EARLY BEGINNINGS
of Anthroposophically
Extended Medicine and
Therapeutic Education
in North America

Early Beginnings

of

Anthroposophically Extended Medicine
and Therapeutic Education
in North America

Compiled by

Bertram von Zabern, MD

Portalbooks ≈ 2024

Portalbooks ≈ 2024

An imprint of SteinerBooks/Anthroposophic Press, Inc.
834 Main Street, PO Box 358, Spencertown, NY 12165
www.SteinerBooks.org

First edition © 2021 Mercury Press

Cover: Weaving designed by Jeanne Ingress, woven by Sirley Reynolds,
Tobias Community, Temple, New Hampshire

LIBRARY OF CONGRESS CONTROL NUMBER: 2024939772

ISBN: 978-1-938685-55-2

Contents

To my parents,

and to my godmother Arvia Mackay-Ege,

who asked me to come to America

Foreword

To devote a book to the remembrance of the pioneers who laid the first foundations of anthroposophically extended medicine and therapeutic education in North America has been a long-standing wish and obligation of mine. Any such reflection contains the question: "Where do we stand today and what is essential for a medicine of true healing?"

Anthroposophically extended medicine, or anthroposophic medicine, is an extension of medicine by the spiritual knowledge of anthroposophy as it was taught by Rudolf Steiner. In their book *Fundamentals for an Extension of the Art of Healing through Spiritual-scientific Knowledge* (translation of its original German title*), Dr. Rudolf Steiner and Dr. Ita Wegman wrote:

> This is not about an opposition against the medicine that works with the acknowledged scientific methods of the present. The latter is fully recognized by us in its principles. And, in our opinion, only one who can be with full validity a physician in the sense of these principles, shall use anthroposophical knowledge in the art of medicine.

---

* This work is currently published as *Extending Practical Medicine: Fundamental Principles Based on the Science of the Spirit* (CW 27), Forest Row, UK: Rudolf Steiner Press, 1997.

Anthroposophic health care professionals have regular training and qualification in their field of practice. In addition, they obtain training based on a view of the whole human being: body, soul, and spirit living in spiritual nature and cosmos. Anthroposophically extended medicine is aware of both the healing treasures of nature and spiritual activity. It uses natural and homeopathic remedies, as well as activating therapies such as eurythmy (creative movement), rhythmical massage, art, and music therapies. Mainstream medication and treatments are included as needed for the benefit of each patient.

An overview in this small format, even if it is limited to the first beginnings made by the founders of anthroposophic medicine and their legacy, cannot be complete and therefore is itself only a beginning. To everyone who so generously contributed to this publication, I want to say a warm, "thank you!" The memories and writings you made available are precious and helpful to us who came later. Special thanks to my wife, Barbara von Zabern, for helping to create this book, to Dr. Alicia Landman-Reiner for editing the 2021 edition, and to the co-workers of SteinerBooks for preparing this new edition.

Bertram von Zabern
Fall 2024

How It Began

In 1920, Rudolf Steiner gave in Dornach, Switzerland, the first course for a wider group of physicians, *Spiritual Science and Medicine*.* One year later the Klinisch-Therapeutische Institut (later named Ita-Wegman Klinik) miraculously came into existence in the neighboring town of Arlesheim. Individually prescribed medicines and remedies (the "Dorons," Iscar, Infludo, etc.) together with a line of body care preparations (Rosemary Soap, Hair Lotion, Ratanhia Mouthwash, etc.) were developed by Dr. Rudolf Steiner, Dr. Ita Wegman, and Dr. Ludwig Noll. They were prepared by chemist Dr. Oskar Schmiedel in a laboratory which quickly grew and received the name of a Druid goddess, Weleda, from Rudolf Steiner in August 1924. It was a time when confidence in the progress of culture had been shattered by both World War I and the global influenza epidemic. A catastrophic breakdown of the world economy was imminent.

Gracia Ricardo, an opera singer, had met Rudolf Steiner and Marie von Sivers (later Marie Steiner) already in 1909 in Berlin. After her return to America in 1910, she became instrumental in forming the first anthroposophical branch in New York City with a unique group of opera singers and artists.

---

* Published as *Introducing Anthroposophical Medicine* (CW 312), Great Barrington, MA: SteinerBooks, 2010.

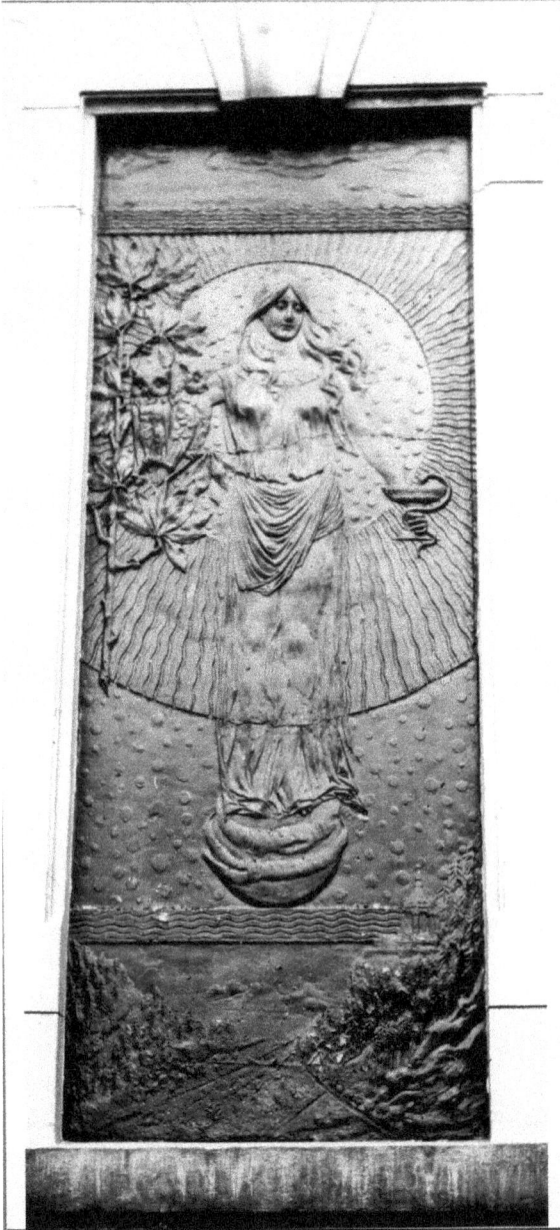

Weleda, at house in Bielefeld, Germany, Gütersloher St. 43a

By the year 1920, the St. Mark Group, which met for years in a studio at Carnegie Hall, had grown to have about thirty members. In Dornach, Rudolf Steiner and Ita Wegman asked Mme. Ricardo if she would be able to get people in America interested in the new remedies. It did not take long for Weleda preparations such as Infludo, Gencydo, and Everon toiletries to be imported and enthusiastically displayed at the Carnegie Hall studio and later in the Threefold Restaurant (which was run by members of the group).

In her classic booklet, *The Earliest Days of Anthroposophy in America,* Hilda Deighton, one of the singers, wrote:

Many of you knew Mme. Ricardo in her later years, as she was active in the American Society in the 1920s and again in the 1940s. When I first met her, she was a majestic and commanding figure. A cosmopolitan personality in the spiritual sense of the word. She had a warrior's bravery, a strong will and a warm heart. When she took a firm stand, she was not easily swayed. She spoke her mind freely and expected others to do the same. When her anger was aroused, it rarely lasted overnight, as she had a forgiving nature and suffered over not always meeting this in others. She tried to begin each day like a clear slate, harboring no ill will. Feeling a deep need for affection herself, she gave it unstintingly to her friends. Her last appearance as a public singer was in 1913 with the pianist Walter Morse Rummel in Berlin, characteristically to raise funds for the building of the first Goetheanum. In the following years she worked toward the development of a new art of tone production fructified by anthroposophy. She returned to New York in 1922 with a special task, that of introducing the anthroposophical medical work to America, an activity she continued long after the organization of the American

Society. Mme. Ricardo spent the rest of her long life interesting people in the works of Rudolf Steiner and teaching singing to a limited number of singers, among whom were Marion Szekely-Freshl, Berty Jenny, Gina Palermo, Mary Theodora Richards and I, all members of the Society. She divided her time between America and Dornach, where she died in 1955.

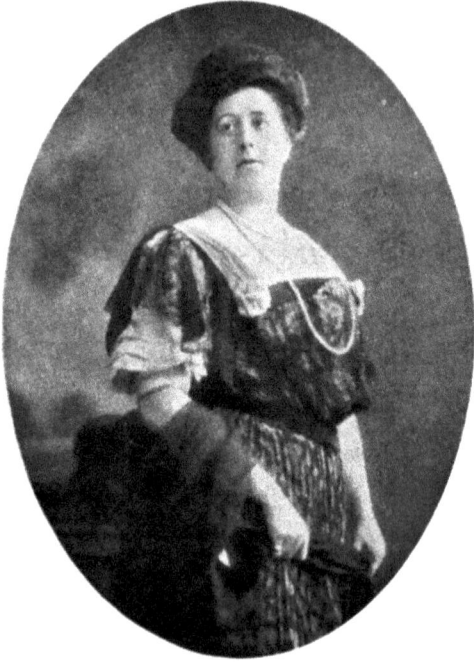

Gracia Ricardo

Among her other initiatives, Mme. Ricardo continued to oversee the importing and distribution of Weleda preparations in America until 1937. There were a growing number of users of the new preparations, which would soon include the patients of Dr. Christoph Linder.

One of the early members of the St. Mark Group, the painter Irene Brown, became a great benefactor of the anthroposophic work happening in New York, especially in the realm of healing. She stayed in Dornach/Arlesheim during 1923/24 to seek treatment for her weak health at the new clinic. In 1924, she brought Lucy van der Pals Neuscheller and her family to New York, as Lucy was invited to teach eurythmy in the beginnings of the first Waldorf school there. Lucy had been trained by the very first eurythmist, Lory Meyer-Smits, in Dornach. In the years to follow, Lucy's initiatives, among them her eurythmy classes, weekly public performances, and the Christmas plays, became an enormous gift to the life of the anthroposophical branch and the therapeutic work taking place there.

Irene Brown was an active force in bringing the first anthroposophic physician to America in 1926. Not only did she fully fund Dr. Linder's move to New York; she made a building at East 39th Street (off Park Avenue) available to anthroposophic initiatives. So, it came about that Dr. Linder's office, Weleda, Mme. Ricardo's residence, and other anthroposophic initiatives were under the same roof for one year! In 1928, the beginnings of the first Waldorf school moved into the same building. The first teachers were Virginia Birdsal, Irene Foltz, Lucy and Leo Neuscheller, and Arvia Mackaye. Sabina Zay (later Nordoff) was among their few students.

In her report, *The History of Weleda USA*, Sophia Christine Molt Murphy describes the following years:

> In 1931, a company was formed for the purpose of importing and distributing Weleda remedies and body care products. It was named Amarlab

(American-Arlesheim Laboratories) and its statutes were signed as trustees by Dr. Ita Wegman, Albert Steffen and Dr. Guenther Wachsmuth for the Goetheanum and Henry B. Monges, Irene Brown, William Scott Pyle and Robert D. Hale, who were leading personalities of the Anthroposophical Society in America. During the early 1930s, Doris Bugby and Arthur von Zabern, the father of Bertram von Zabern, M.D., worked at Weleda/Amarlab for several years (Arthur returned in 1932 to Europe to devote his life's work to Weleda). In 1937, Walter Molt came from Stuttgart to take on the directorship of Amarlab from Mme. Ricardo.

Dr. Christoph Linder (1897–1964)

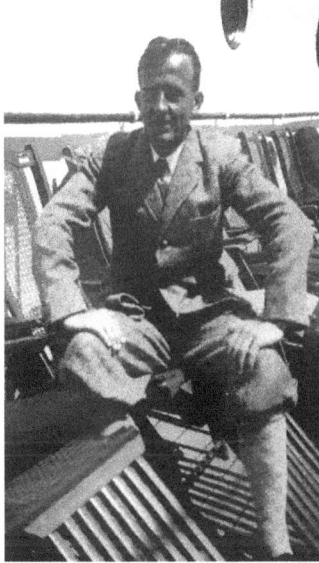

Henry Barnes, who had known Dr. Linder through many years, wrote in his book *Into the Heart's Land*:

> The first physician to practice anthroposophically extended medicine was Christoph Linder, MD. He was born in Basel, Switzerland, on January 26, 1897, as the fourth child of a well-to-do family. From the age of fourteen Christoph knew that he wanted to be a doctor. He attended high school in Basel and went to medical studies at Lausanne. After receiving his medical degree, he fulfilled his internship and residency in Frankfurt am Main. He encountered anthroposophy and not only heard Rudolf

Steiner speak at the Goetheanum, but also met him personally. In 1925, he was studying anthroposophically extended medicine and working at the clinic in Arlesheim under Dr. Wegman's direction, when he was invited to the United States by Irene Brown. Christoph's older brother was then living and working as a banker in New York City, when Christoph paid his first visit to this country. He was considering joining Albert Schweitzer in Africa when Ita Wegman asked whether he would go to New York to establish the anthroposophical medical work. This was, again, at the invitation and urging of Irene Brown. He hesitated for some time, but finally decided to accept the invitation. He moved to New York in 1926.

There, he opened his office in the same building at East 39th Street, where the Rudolf Steiner School would open its doors in 1928 and where Mme. Gracia Ricardo lived and worked for the sale and distribution of Weleda products. As we already know, this was the building that Irene Brown had bought and placed at the service of anthroposophy.

Dr. Linder was primarily affiliated with the Flower-Fifth Avenue Hospital. He also served as the official physician of the Swiss consulate in New York City, and as a member of the Swiss Benevolent Association. He was also the school doctor for the Rudolf Steiner School for many years.

From the beginning of the 1950s, Dr. Linder, a general internist, held meetings at his house for doctors, pharmacists, researchers, and specifically medically interested individuals. These meetings were held quarterly for the most part. Katherine Brydert, MD, an obstetrician, was a faithful attendee. Franz Winkler, MD, a well-known internist in New York City, participated, as did Henry Williams, MD, from Lancaster, Pennsylvania. The faithful pharmacist Ernst

Schiller, who carried the Weleda pharmaceutical work at the Goodman Pharmacy, was frequently there. Anna Koffler (later Wannamaker), a medicinal

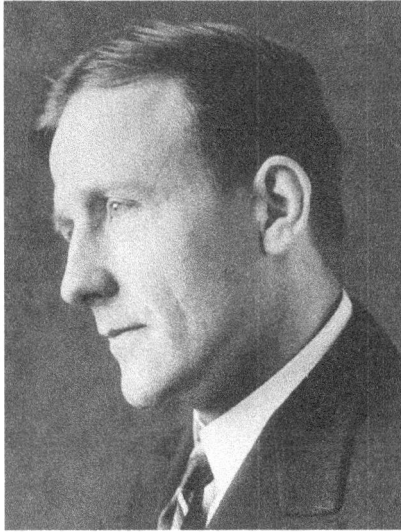

Dr. Linder in 1933

herbalist, attended occasionally. The biochemical researcher, Ehrenfried Pfeiffer, MD hon., attended at intervals. Karl Ernst Schaefer, MD, who was in charge of physiological research at the submarine base in New London, Connecticut, would join in to share his perspectives. Howard Laskey, MD, from Rhode Island, took part on occasion. By the mid-fifties, Paul Scharff, MD, and Ursula Weber, MD, joined in regularly. By this time, Sigfrid Knauer, MD, was established in California and Traute Page, MD, was practicing in Chicago. Neither Dr. Knauer nor Dr. Page joined these meetings at this time, although Dr. Page took part at a later time.

During most of the 1950s this same group formed the nucleus for science conferences that took place at the initiative of Ehrenfried Pfeiffer at the Threefold

Farm at Spring Valley, New York, and occasionally elsewhere. Christoph Linder was a regular participant at these conferences, as well as at the summer school conferences sponsored by the Spiritual Science Foundation (which later became the Threefold Education Foundation). The first of the summer conferences was held in July 1933 at the Threefold Farm.

It was also during the middle years of the 1950s that a group of interested individuals gathered around Christoph Linder to form the Fellowship Committee within the Anthroposophical Society. The Committee came into existence because of the needs of some older members. It was this initiative that eventually led to the establishment of the Fellowship Community in Spring Valley, New York.

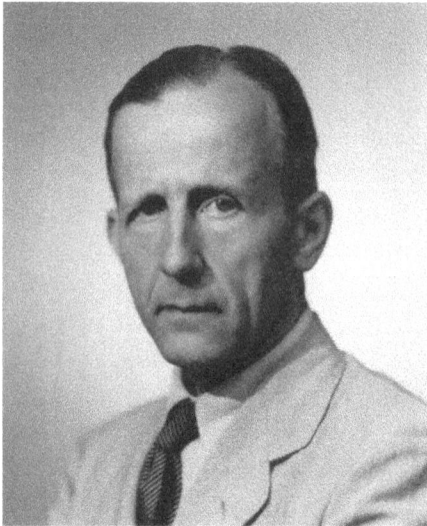

Dr. Linder in 1950

Dr. Maria C. Linder (Dr. Linder's daughter, who was a professor of biochemistry and on the active staff of the California State University in Fullerton) wrote in support of this commemoration:

> Dr. Linder was a very kind and caring person, though his face was a bit stoic and some people did at times mistake it as meaning he was very serious. In meeting someone he would certainly have gone towards them and shaken their hand. He was a very patient man, and also very calm in the face of a crisis. I remember how reassuring that was when I fell from riding the banisters in our five-story house and cut into my tongue, releasing lots of blood. He was so calm, and it made a great deal of difference. He also went out of his way to make visitors from Europe or my sisters and my friends welcome in our house in New York— for meals or to invite them to our house in the country.
>
> He was someone with deep integrity and for whom the truth was the most important thing. Yet it was also okay to make mistakes as long as we learned from them. He truly cared for others, and he was always very generous—with his time, his attention (he spent lots of time with each patient), and helped out those who were less well-off for all kinds of reasons. He treated many people without expecting payment or for a very low fee. We often visited patients—especially farmers, on our way to the country, and he might get a good loaf of bread in return.
>
> My father loved to take walks and hikes. In the country we would do lots of walks in the forests and along paths, and go swimming in a lake that was nearby. In Switzerland he loved to walk in the mountains with us (and our big family over there), and also did a few alpine glacier climbs. He even liked to plant things, especially fruit trees, and tend to them, working in

the garden. In the city, we often went to museums as well as take walks in Central Park, to the zoo, and to occasional concerts (classical) and/or anthroposophic events.

My parents married in Dornach, Switzerland in 1937, in the presence of Albert Steffen, right by the Goetheanum. Afterwards they traveled by ship to New York. My mother, Maria Ruth Philippi Linder, was a eurythmist at the Goetheanum from 1933 to 1937, and took part in many stage performances. She died in 1957.

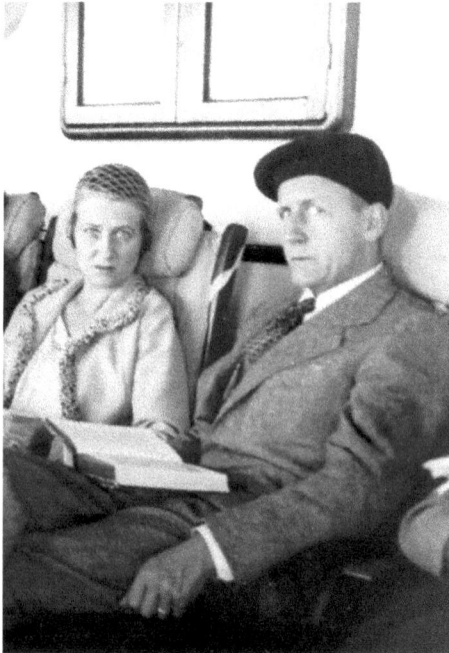

Ruth and Christoph Linder on their passage to New York in 1937

In his Christoph Linder Memorial Lecture given in February 1966, we heard Dr. Winkler's words:

I shall stress the two qualities which, in more than twenty years of friendship with Dr. Christoph Linder, I came to admire most. I hope that you in your hearts will join me in this commemoration and add other cherished memories of your own. His two dominant traits were his longing to heal rather than to treat, and his unwavering determination to carry out what he considered to be right. The latter, this almost stubborn determination, is rare indeed. A little soul searching, if done in earnest, will quickly dispel some of our favorite illusions. It will show only too often how all of us find reasons to deviate from a course of action which deep in our hearts we know is right. Christoph, as any other human being, may at times have been mistaken about the right or wrong choice. Yet unlike so many others, he individually tried to do what he considered to be right.

Christoph Linder suffered a disabling stroke in 1961. After seeking treatment at the Clinic in Arlesheim, he returned to New York where he remarried. "Anita Nef Linder, was the closest to Christoph at the most crucial period of his life and was primarily responsible for turning a year of torment into a year of inner victory" (Franz Winkler in his lecture, above). Paul Scharff said, "He died as a master." Dr. Linder had asked Dr. Scharff to continue the mission given to him by Ita Wegman.

More Pioneer Years of Weleda

Sophia Christine Molt Murphy, Walter Molt's daughter, wrote:

In 1937, Walter Molt came over from Germany to become the managing director of Amarlab. Within a few months of his arrival, he changed the name of the corporation to Weleda. In the beginning of World War II, Walter Molt stockpiled Weleda ingredients and medicines, foreseeing that the import from Europe might become impossible. He also built a relationship with Dr. Ehrenfried Pfeiffer who had been developing biodynamic methods of gardening and farming. Pfeiffer was glad to plant medicinal herbs for Weleda at the Myrin Farm in Kimberton, Pennsylvania (now Camphill, Kimberton Hills). Because of these precautions the company was able to supply for most needs during the war years.

In 1939, Dr. Ernst Schiller arrived in New York, an Austrian pharmacist who had fled the Nazi regime. Walter Molt employed him recognizing his special qualities, and Schiller cared for the medicine preparation for the next thirty-five years. A friend of Ernst Schiller, Dr. Clara Fürst also joined. She was, like Dr. Schiller, a pharmacist from Austria and became a faithful helper.

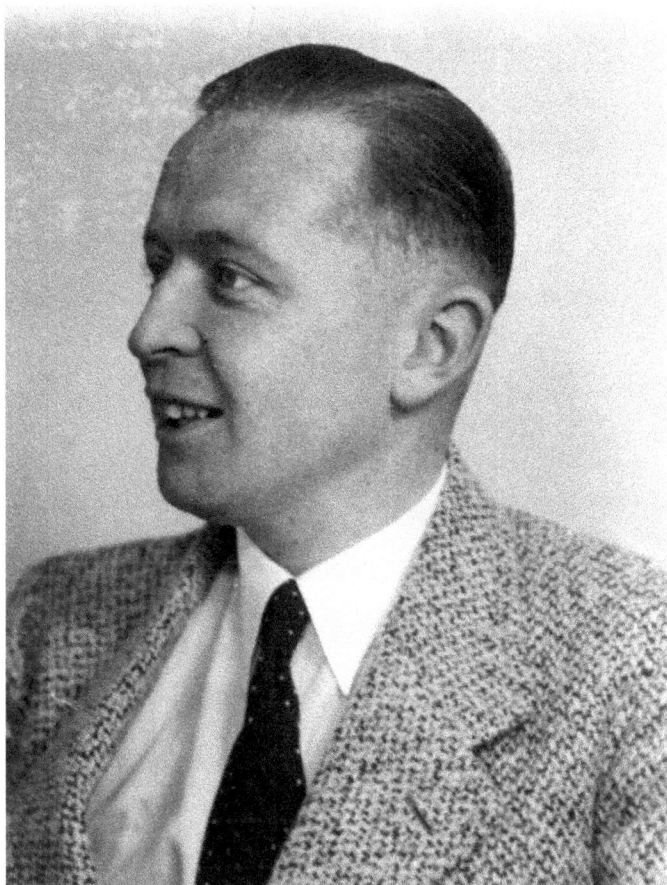

Walter Molt (1906–1974)

In her book, *The Multifaceted Life of Emil Molt (Founder of the Waldorf School)*, Sophia Christine shares the drama of the new family's emigration to America:

> After Emil Molt's funeral, Edgar Dürler, who had come from the Swiss Weleda, paid a visit to Walter asking him whether he would be willing to manage the Austrian Weleda. Walter said he'd love to work for Weleda, but had no inclination to stay in a National

Socialist country, upon which Dürler mentioned the tiny Weleda in New York needed a director.

In the first days of January 1937, when I was ten days old, Walter crossed the Swiss border on the pretext that he had accounts to settle for his father. From there he went to France and boarded a ship for America. He was now classed a traitor to his country. For three months my mother, now classed as the wife of a deserter, tried in vain to obtain a visa. She was lucky. On one day her search took her to an official whose child's life had been saved by her father. Out of gratitude and against all protocol, this man handed her an exit visa.

In a recent letter, Sophia Christine describes her father as a sensitive and warmhearted person who was at times over-burdened by the pioneer situation of the American Weleda.

Walter was born in 1906, the only child of Berta and Emil Molt. His father was an industrialist and became the founder of the first Waldorf school. Rudolf Steiner was often a guest of the Molt family in Stuttgart. Walter's cousin, Lisa Dreher Monges, told that as a guest, Rudolf Steiner loved to entertain the children. He would tell them stories and show them little tricks, one being how to cut an apple in such a way that it held together in one piece. The children would then be surprised, suddenly seeing that the apple had two pieces. Meeting Rudolf Steiner as a child and as a young man both in his family life and in the Waldorf School was deeply formative for Walter. He grew up as his father's helper in times of crisis. Later, he had the foresight to bring his young family to safety in the United States and to steer the fledgling American Weleda through World War II and the postwar years.

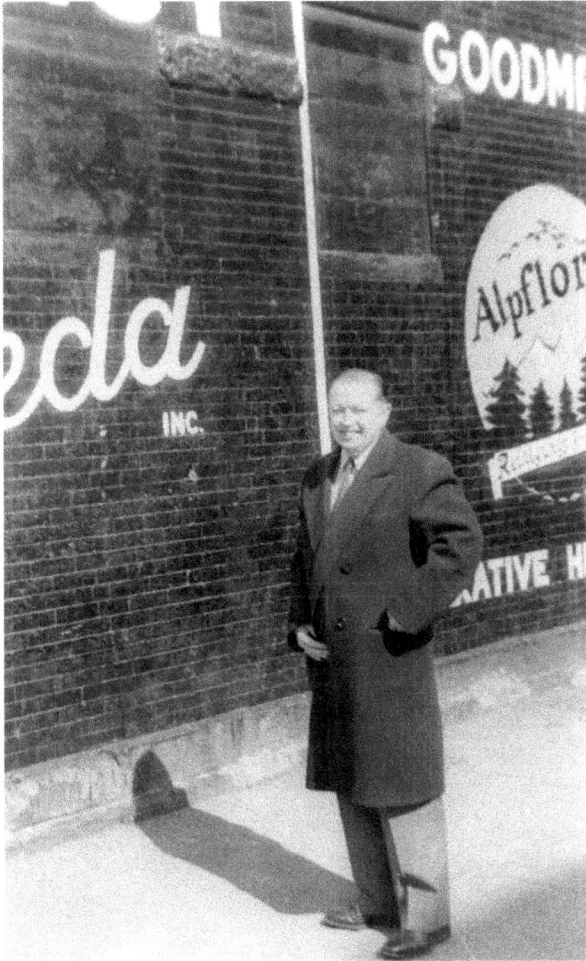

Walter

Walter and Edith had married in 1934. Christine was born shortly before the emigration of the young family, which soon grew with the arrival of the younger sister, Ursula. In the years to come they lived mostly at the Threefold Farm Community in Spring Valley, a short trip out of New York City. First Dr. Linder, later Dr. Winkler were their family doctors, both remembered as gentle, perceptive, and gentlemanly. After twenty-eight years, Walter handed

Weleda (which had considerably grown and was then located at Goodman's Pharmacy) to Sophia Christine and her husband Finbarr Murphy in early 1965. The Molts retired to southern Switzerland, where they fixed up an old house in a village overlooking Lago Maggiore. They helped a local Waldorf school and, remarkably, invited thalidomide children to their house for their holidays. Walter reached the age of sixty-eight, Edith the age of eighty-three.

Here is Dr. Ernst Schiller's description of the pioneer years, which was kindly provided by Sophia Christine:

> My own knowledge about Weleda, New York dates from the day on which I first met Walter Molt in February of 1939. What I knew at that time about the activities and the purpose of the Weleda Company in Europe resulted from my reading the *Weleda Nachrichten* (Weleda News), a publication we received regularly at the pharmacy in Vienna, where I had been employed for several years. Without that cursory information I would most likely not have applied for the job, when I heard by chance that Mr. Molt was looking for a pharmacist. The company was at that time established in the rooms in a loft on Fourth Avenue at 19th Street. The equipment consisted (aside from the office) of some steel shelving, a small pony mixer, an ointment mill, a gas burner, and a sink with cold and hot water faucets.
>
> All the medicinal items were imported from Arlesheim in half and one-ounce bottles, ready to be dispensed. In New York there were two pharmacies, which carried our products before I arrived. A few products, which could be sold over the counter, like Pine Bath, Rosemary Bath, Birch Syrup, and a few cosmetic preparations, like Skin Cream, Cold Cream, Dental Lotion (now called Mouth Wash), and a dental

cream, were made here with the assistance of a chemist who had his own small establishment on the same floor. He probably was an able chemist, and I learned a few things from him. But he could not give us much of his time and gradually it became evident that improvements were in order. Also, the enactment of the new drug laws made it inevitable to acquire a pharmacy license, and I was hired with this in mind.

At first, I restricted my activity to improving the quality of those preparations that had already been introduced into the market. Their shelf life had to be prolonged because turnover was still slow. Bottles of Birch preparation used to explode, bath emulsions separated, etc. The only technical information about Weleda products and instructions for their manufacture came from a notebook that Mr. Molt had brought with him (I believe that this "Black Book" must still be around somewhere). This I had to supplement with my own experience as a pharmacist and some advice from the aforementioned neighbor chemist (airmail had only recently been established and therefore communications with the parent company in Europe were slow and scanty. It was only after the war, in 1950, that I was sent to Arlesheim and Schwäbisch Gmünd for several weeks of intensive training).

When it became evident that America would enter the war in Europe, we ordered a large supply of preparations in concentrated form (mother tinctures and low potencies, which I could turn into finished products ready to be distributed) from our parent company. In time, more and more preparations could be made here, especially after we moved to larger and better equipped quarters on West 57th Street, on the same floor as the Anthroposophical Society and Press. For me these were the best accommodations we ever had.

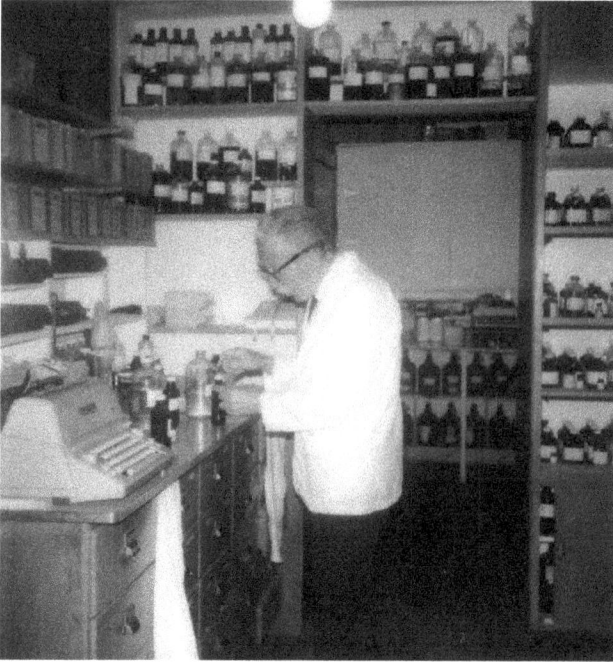

Dr. Ernst Schiller

One day, after I had obtained my license, I visited Dr. Clara Fürst, a pharmacist and chemist who had been an apprentice in the store where I was employed in Vienna. She worked in a chemical laboratory in a building next to where we were. It turned out that she was not very happy there, and I suggested to Mr. Molt that he hire her as my assistant. He did, which turned out to be a very lucky move. Dr. Fürst stayed with us for many years making ampules, a very exacting and tedious operation which we later discontinued. She worked mostly in the office, where her fabulous memory was a valuable asset. She knew payment records by heart, no need to consult books!

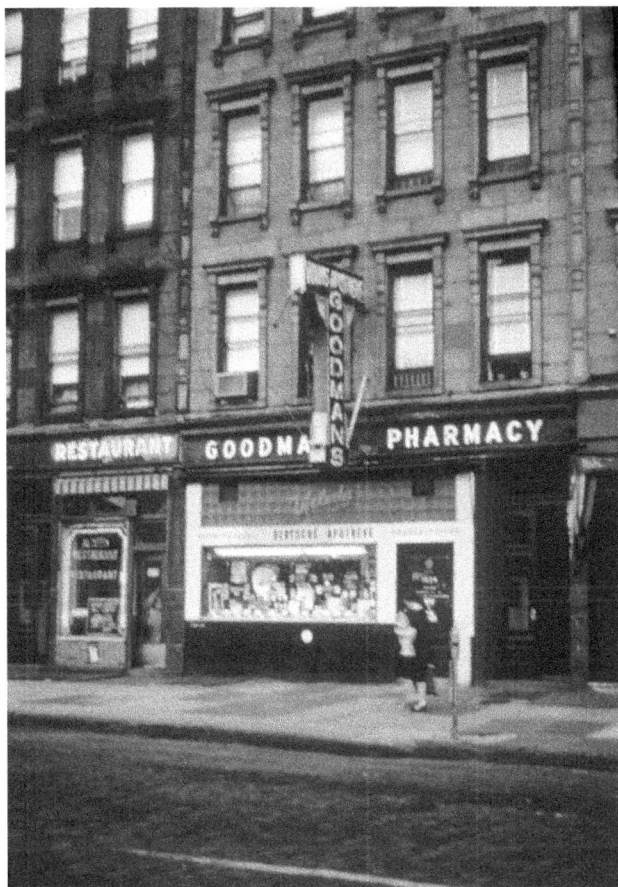

When the headquarters of the Society and press were moved to their present location on Madison Avenue, we could not move along with them because of zoning regulations. Mr. Molt found premises for us on Broadway near 82nd Street and furnished them nicely for us. He had a special knack for planning and executing such moves. About a year later, when I came back from a vacation in Maine, I learned that Mr. Molt had bought the Goodman Pharmacy on First Avenue in Yorkville. I was stunned, because never before had Walter Molt made a decision so suddenly. At first, I did not like the idea at all, because I was determined not to go into the retail pharmacy business in this country. After the war had ended, the Goodman Pharmacy flourished because the Germans in Yorkville bought everything to send to their relatives in the old country.

As an institution, the Goodman Pharmacy was interesting and fascinating. Mr. Goodman, its founder, operated it to satisfy his ambition to be a healer and benefactor (he made his money elsewhere, in real estate). To this purpose he had built up a stock of herbs as complete as any I have ever seen. Popular items like peppermint leaves and chamomile flowers were bought from a reputable wholesaler, and there were hundreds of different kinds. These herbs were combined in ten mixtures that were supposed to cure specific ailments like rheumatism, colds, stomach trouble, constipation, obesity, etc. From these herbs and some simple harmless chemicals he devised clever and effective formulae for preparations in various forms, such as fluids, powders, tablets, suppositories, ointments, and injectables that sold throughout the country. At the time when he sold his enterprise to Weleda (at a very reasonable price), the new drug laws and restrictions became effective and such practices were gradually made impossible. But for a number of years, we were able to profit from the reputation of the store on a somewhat limited scale.

So far, I have not mentioned that the wellbeing—actually the very existence of Weleda—depended on the presence of a sufficient number of anthroposophic physicians who created the demand for our products. In 1939, there were only two such ones in New York City, one in Wyoming, and two others. In 1940, Dr. Winkler came and, along with Dr. Linder, kept us fairly busy. For a number of years Dr. Laskey in Rhode

Island kept us very busy. He had come to anthroposophic medicine by way of veterinary prescriptions and via biodynamic gardening and farming. He was very eager to use our remedies but was limited by lack of literature in English. Dr. Karl Ernst Schaefer lived in his vicinity and he could communicate with him. It was a great loss when Dr. Linder died quite early and Dr. Winkler a few years later.

When Dr. Scharff established his office in Spring Valley, New York, and the community there began to grow, Mr. Murphy suggested moving the Weleda to Spring Valley. He was never very happy about the association between Weleda and Goodman Pharmacy. So, when the public interest in the latter began to decline, he found the time ripe for a move.

Thanks to the interest of a number of anthroposophic physicians and a few outsiders, Weleda is now able to stand on its own legs with just some minor support from Europe. Our main purpose is still to supply remedies for the ailing, but we also need the support of our healthy friends we serve.

After Weleda had found a new home at the Threefold and Fellowship communities in Spring Valley (now Chestnut Ridge), New York, a considerable hurdle had to be overcome. Due to the growing health-food market and increased demand for body-care products Weleda's production had increased. But stricter regulations by the Food and Drug Administration could only be met after a breakthrough deal was reached in 1988 in close collaboration with the homeopathic community. The Homeopathic Pharmacopeia (HPUS) became the regulatory body for medicine preparation and distribution. The distribution of remedies imported from Europe, also prepared at their own compound pharmacy, increased considerably through the presence of new anthro-posophic physicians. In 1994, the ownership of Weleda USA was handed over to the parent company in Switzerland.

Finbarr and Sophia Christine stayed for a number of years to ensure an optimal transition. They retired in 2002 to Ireland, Finbarr's native country. Since then, the company's home continued to be in upstate New York. In 2012 the company moved to Irvington, New York, a short way from New York City, where it all began a century ago.

Dr. Franz E. Winkler (1907–1972)

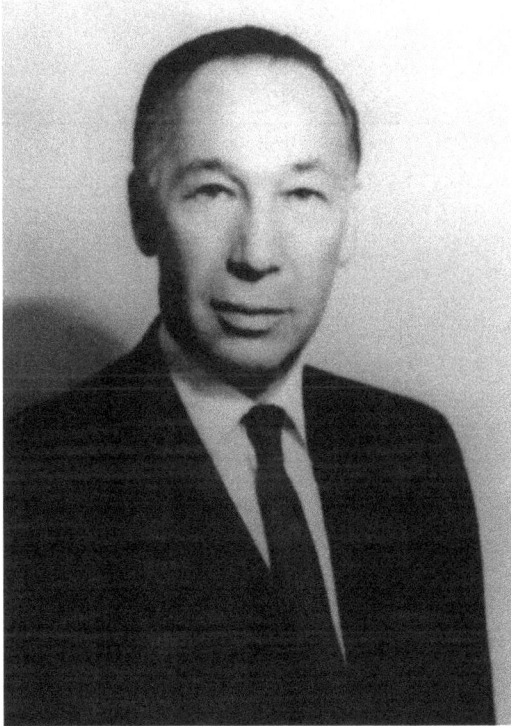

The following commemoration was given by Dr. George K. Russell, professor emeritus of biology at Adelphi University:

> Franz E. Winkler was born in Vienna in 1907. His childhood was profoundly affected by the first World War, and it was a time of great struggle and privation for his family. Following the war, he completed

his schooling and entered medical college, and in 1932 he was awarded the MD degree by the University of Vienna. Among his teachers and associates were such notables as Alfred Adler, Sigmund Freud, Viktor Frankl, Karl König and the Nobel laureate, Julius Wagner-Jauregg. As a young doctor he had occasion to examine some of Freud's patients and had highly interesting comments to make about them. Early in his career he was appointed head physician at a private hospital for psychological and neurological diseases in Rekawinkel. But the German annexation of Austria in March 1938 radically changed the course of his life and, together with his wife Dorothea Weiss Winkler, he left Europe for the United States. They were among the last to leave Austria before the borders were slammed shut by the Nazis.

After qualifying in the U.S., Franz Winkler established a medical practice in New York and continued his work there until his death at the age of sixty-four. His patients included a number of well-known figures in public life and many typical American families who entrusted themselves to his care, often for decades. It was his conviction that it was the physician's task, and opportunity, to befriend his patients and to be able to assess a patient's state of physical and psychological wellbeing over long periods of time, especially during the crucial periods of adolescence as well as in adult life with its challenges and tribulations. He often reflected on the state of affairs in the world through the lens of his own patients and their problems.

A central feature of his approach was to see that physical illnesses often mirrored the inner state of the patient. In his view, fundamental causes frequently lay in the person's inner psychological life, and the outer manifestations, symptomatically, were the wide variety of physical ailments he saw in the medical office. He looked in other cases for the roots of mental afflictions in organically based disorders. The contrast between physical conditions with psychological causes and mental afflictions with physical causes was of the greatest interest to him and such considerations formed one of the foundation stones of his practice. With deeply rooted illnesses of the psyche, he knew that the physician is obliged to prescribe a wide variety of pharmacological agents and medical treatments, but, additionally, he must help the patient gain insights into his own psyche, so to speak, and work to bring restorative measures and balance to his inner life.

True healing, Dr. Winkler often stated, begins with genuine self-knowledge and a firm determination to address and work assiduously on matters in the realm of the psyche. In this way, the overcoming of illness becomes a challenge and opportunity for inner growth and personal development. Franz Winkler practiced a unique brand of medicine that included the wealth of medications and treatments derived from anthroposophical medicine and the work of Dr. Rudolf Steiner, many of the developments of modern allopathic medicine, and his own extraordinary gifts of compassion and medical intuition.

From his earliest days in the United States, Dr. Winkler gave public lectures on a wide variety of topics, such as the future of medicine, the role of America in world affairs, the true nature of human freedom, educational reforms, and the dangers of mind-altering substances. He also placed great hopes in the Waldorf school movement, and he served as medical consultant to several of these schools. In the young people who came his way he hoped to find leaders for the future—that is, individuals who could bring imaginative and creative solutions to the problems of modern life. It was his conviction that the pedagogical methods used in Waldorf schools helped greatly to prepare individuals who could meet the challenges of our times with courage, imagination, and genuine idealism.

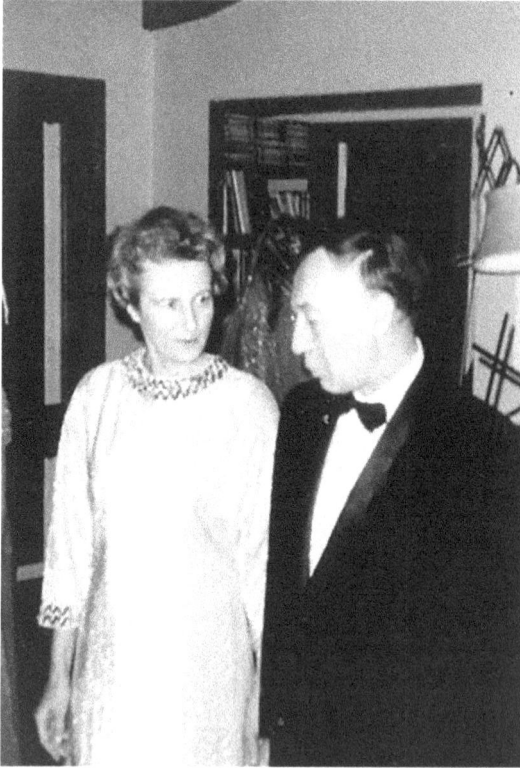

Dorothea and Franz Winkler

Franz Winkler had a deep commitment to the protection of animal life and to the conservation movement as a whole. He welcomed the Wilderness Act of 1964 as an extremely important contribution to the collective health and wellbeing of the country, and he wrote letters to the Canadian government on behalf of the Atlantic fur seals in the St. Lawrence River. In a personal notebook discovered after his death there was a listing of animal causes he wished to support. He wrote that the kinds of animal experiments (vivisections and dissections) often conducted in high schools and colleges teach nothing but cruelty, and he was opposed to any sort of animal suffering in the name of education. He urged the use of anatomical models rather than animal specimens in teaching, and he encouraged teachers to help their students learn to observe and study living animals in their natural environment. He was also aware of the nature of animal slaughter, and he favored the development of more humane slaughter methods and their strict enforcement.

In the mid-1950s he decided that further efforts were needed to bring important thoughts to the American public, so together with Mr. H.A.W. Myrin he founded The Myrin Institute, a private operating foundation dedicated to a renewal of culture and to a new understanding of modern life and its many problems. For many years Myrin published a series of pamphlets, the "Myrin Institute Proceedings," and the following list reflects a small sampling of the topics and authors whose thoughts contributed to this effort: "National Psychology in International Relations," by Franz E. Winkler; "The Experience of Knowledge," by John F. Gardner; "The Scientific and Moral in Education," by Francis Edmunds; "Intellect, Intuition, and the Racial Question," by Laurens van der Post; "Pollution of the I," by Jacques Lusseyran; "The Role of Technology in the Modern World," by Frederick Kreitner; "American Indians and Our Way of Life," by Sylvester Morey; "Marijuana Today," by George K. Russell; "The Secret of Peace and The Environmental Crisis," by John F. Gardner; and numerous others. These monographs found their way into American life and brought many individuals into contact with the Myrin Institute. Following Dr. Winkler's death, Myrin continued its work and has made significant contributions to contemporary life. These efforts include a decades-long effort in the field of substance abuse and the establishment of a subsidiary organization, the American Council for Drug Education. Through conferences, publications, and other means the ACDE (now a branch of Phoenix House in New York) has brought the dangers of mind-altering drugs to a wide audience. And in 1982, Myrin founded *Orion* magazine, later to be incorporated into the Orion Society. The magazine continues today and aims to bring a broad range of environmental matters to the attention of its readers. A principal theme is the ongoing effort to remind readers that direct experience of nature is a source of true motivation for the protection of the natural environment. Franz Winkler often reminded those who came to his office or attended one of his lectures that we will protect and defend with determination and enthusiasm what we have come to love and admire.

Perhaps Franz Winkler's greatest achievement was his influential book, *Man: The Bridge Between Two Worlds*, published by Harper and Row in 1960. In this volume, Dr. Winkler addresses a wide variety of practical and philosophical questions. Surely the most important of these is the question of cognition. How do we know what we know? Put somewhat differently, how do we arrive at truth? Is it only through the empirical methods of scientific analysis, or is there an additional pathway to knowledge and deeper understanding? His answer is clearly articulated in the book. Knowing is twofold, he asserts. It combines *intellectual* analysis with what he terms *intuitive* understanding—i.e., a faculty for comprehending that we all possess but is far less developed and very poorly understood.

In a notable passage he writes, "One of the most far-reaching mistakes of present-day thinking is to assume that comprehension is a result of intellectual effort. Intellect is descriptive and differentiating; it classifies and orders; it informs us of the mechanics of natural and even spiritual processes, but it does not help us understand their true nature. Of course, intellect is needed for cognition. For thanks to its analytical power, it is capable of splitting complex phenomena into their integral parts that must be studied as individual entities. But, if unchecked by the synthesizing faculty of intuition, analysis will continue until the unifying principle is lost in a maze of incomprehensible facts."

Dr. Winkler's theme of intuition is fully developed in *Man: The Bridge*, and one of the final chapters bears the compelling title "Training in Intuition." Through developed and trained intuition, he writes, the individual can come to deep insights regarding the great cosmic questions of life and can develop a true understanding of intangibles such as love, freedom, and the nature of the human spirit. In his view, the greatest need of modern human beings is a reconciliation of the findings of modern science with a spiritual view of life. Trained intuition, he writes, offers that possibility. He often argued that no single fact of science, provided that it is a genuine fact, can contradict a spiritual conception of life. *Man: The Bridge Between Two Worlds* has influenced many readers. And for those individuals earnestly seeking answers to the fundamental questions of existence, Franz Winkler's thesis offers, shall we say, genuine food for thought.

Franz Winkler was also deeply interested in myths, legends, and fairytales. He held that such fables and tales, originating from much older times, were based on the intuitive consciousness of earlier peoples who, like young children, were less intellectual and far more intuitive. Myths of all sorts, he often stated,

give powerful insights into the human condition and
into life itself. Out of a deep love of music and his
lifelong interest in myth, Franz Winkler gave a series
of public lectures on mythology in Richard Wagner's
Ring series. These were printed individually and then
compiled into a single volume, published as *For Freedom Destined: Mysteries of Man's Evolution in the
Mythology of Wagner's Ring Operas and Parsifal.*

It is my hope that readers who find value in this
short sketch of Franz Winkler's lifework will wish to
read further in the body of his published work. His
writings, I am convinced, bring a bright light to a
world that is growing ever darker. A listing of his published works is available at www.myrin.org.

Mrs. Jeanne Hawthorne, who was a patient of Dr. Winkler,
remembers:

Franz Winkler entered the life of my family at the end
of summer 1950. I was fourteen years old and about to
enter the freshman year at High Mowing School. We
were directed toward Franz when, as we were told, he
would be one who would be able to see and correct a
condition my father had that, if not corrected, would
end his life prematurely.

Franz, through a twenty-year period, became
friend, father figure, mentor, and guide. His gentleness,
humor, wisdom, and caring for us made visits to him
a joy and an adventure. Relationships were smoothed
out among family members, friends, and colleagues at
work. The path of my own life always seemed to be
now on a more certain course. The example he set for
me, out of himself, touched me deeply.

I will not forget the little story he told us at our
first meeting around that dining table in Spring Valley in 1950. In his quiet way, he told us about an

incident at his family home in Austria when he was a boy. In those days, salesmen would come to your home carrying their wares. One day, a salesman came to the house carrying baskets of tomatoes. He knocked on the doors; there were two front doors. The doors, after a moment or two, began to open. They opened, opened, and opened very slowly and quietly. But no person was in sight. The family, at this particular time, were away but also a part of the family were two dogs. The dogs knew how to open these two front doors! When the family returned home later, tomatoes were everywhere. Not a salesman was in sight. There was quite a mess to clean up, and those dogs did look a bit guilty!

We four young ones, one young one and three children, loved this story. Franz became a very dear friend and trusted physician. My father's condition was corrected and our other physical ailments carefully watched over, doors to the wider world opened, and by example and with suggestions he gave to us ways in which we could, and should, embrace this world, ourselves, and our paths. These legacies he left us.

Franz did—with a bit of scolding, for I was someone who favored our anthroposophic medications only—say to me that if a person who really wished to heal other human beings had the chance to create a medication, that medication would have in it that strong wish to heal, and heal.

David W. White, an alumnus of the Garden City and High Mowing Waldorf schools, contributed:

Dr. Winkler was the medical advisor to the Garden City Waldorf School until the time of his death and served on their advisory board. Mr. Alarik Myrin, who had put up the funds to start the school in 1947, first met

Dr. Winkler that year. It was to Dr. Winkler that Mr. Myrin turned the following year when the young school was having difficulties, and from 1949 on the tide at the school turned to a more flourishing evolution.

Dr. Winkler became physician and friend to many teachers, parents, and children and was always ready to give the right advice at the right time. He seemed to sense the best in human beings and showed them how to bring that forth. Dr. Winkler also served on the first board of trustees at High Mowing—through 1965 or so, I believe. There, he was also a friend and guide to many.

Dr. Sigfrid Knauer (1894–1984)

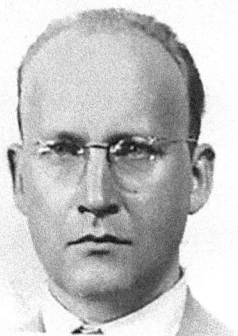

Dr. Sigfrid Knauer.

Sigfrid Knauer was born in Kiev, Ukraine, the son of a professor of languages at the Kiev University. He grew up with his brother and four sisters, all of whom became connected to anthroposophy. His sister Ilse was well known as an anthroposophic ophthalmologist who developed therapeutic eurythmy for eye conditions.* Sigfrid studied medicine and received his medical degree in 1919 in Jena, Germany. As a medical student, not having yet heard about anthroposophy, he wrote an essay, *The Significance of Man's Upright Position*, which earned him the first prize.

Having participated in the Young Doctors' Course** and other medical courses given by Rudolf Steiner, he was

---

* See Daniela Armstrong and Ilse Knauer, *Therapeutic Eurythmy for the Eyes,* Chestnut Ridge, NY: Mercury Press, 2020.

** Published as *Understanding Healing: Meditative Reflections on Deepening Medicine through Spiritual Science* (CW 316), Forest Row, UK: Rudolf Steiner Press 2013.

advised by him to go into the field of cancer research. In the 1930s, Dr. Knauer had his practice for a number of years in Berlin. He soon gained a reputation for his approach to cancer. He was a family doctor and the school physician for the Berlin Waldorf School. Sigfrid and his wife, Edith, wanted no part of the Nazi regime. With the help of Olin Wannamaker, a leading American anthroposophist, the family emigrated in 1939 to the United States shortly before the borders were closed.

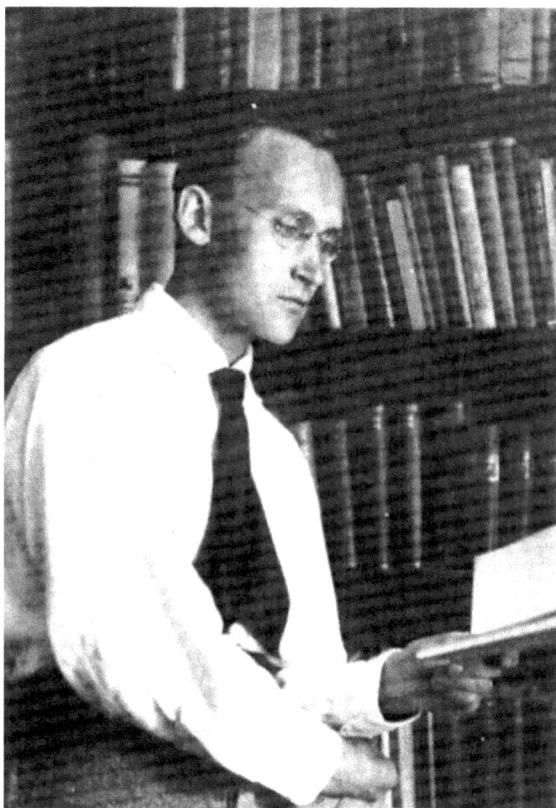

Finding it difficult to obtain a license in New York, Dr. Knauer and his family moved to Los Angeles, where he became licensed as a physician. Soon, he opened his practice on Sunset Boulevard in Hollywood. Though the office space was small, the location was prominent. It was said that Dr. Knauer's patients came from all avenues of life, but celebrities from arts and film found their way to his office and were seen in conversation while waiting (sometimes for hours) to be seen by the doctor. Dr. Knauer's personality was immediately comforting to many patients. By the time a thorough consultation was finished, he would select the right remedy for the patient from his huge collection of homeopathic preparations. Such a collection was necessary, especially during and after the war, when medication shipments from Europe and even from New York City took a very long time.

Sigfrid and Edith were active members of the anthroposophical branch in Los Angeles. His lectures drew large audiences. One member said, "There was nothing usual about him; people either totally go for him, or they completely disagree." Dr. Knauer was the school physician at the Highland Hall School for many years while it was the only Waldorf school in the American West.

Tragedy struck when Edith, the mother of their four children, died of cancer in 1948. In 1953, Sigfrid was married to Indra Devi, with whom he remained together until the end of his life. She was born in Riga, Latvia, which was at that time part of the tsarist empire, like Ukraine. They met at his office and discovered they could both speak Russian, the language familiar to both since childhood. The similar paths walked in their early lives made it easy for them to forge their bond. Indra was an internationally known yoga teacher who introduced yoga as a therapeutic and recreational element to many people's lives in America through her classes and books. She had become particularly popular among Hollywood celebrities. In 1961, Sigfrid helped to purchase a farm retreat near Tecate, Mexico, close to the American border. Indra gave many yoga classes there for years.

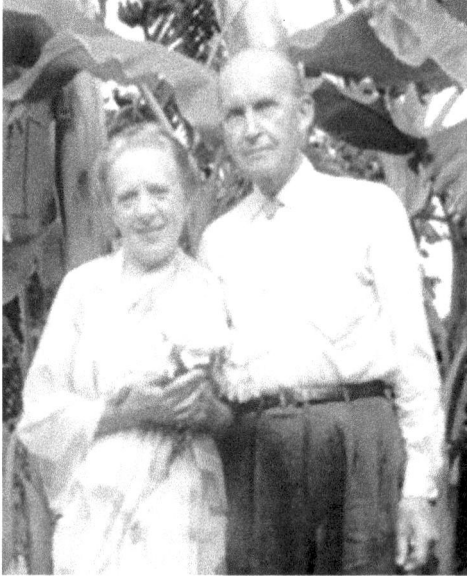

Indra Devi and Sigfrid Knauer

By the mid-1970s, medical regulations in California had become more stringent. Dr. Knauer realized his practice there would become too limited. He decided to move his office to the retreat across the Mexican border. On one of these trips he had a car accident, followed by a stroke. After suffering a second, even more severe stroke and being hospitalized, a group of his friends and patients created a setting for his recovery near Sacramento. In 1980, part of his care came from Dr. Christina (Christa) van Tellingen and her husband Hendrik, a physiotherapist. One of Sigfrid's daughters visited frequently. Now himself a patient, a new aspect of Dr. Knauer's individuality came forth and inspired many around him. It took more than a year before he regained some strength and mobility. It was likely in 1981 that he left California, having been the only anthroposophic physician in the North American West for more than forty years. He joined his wife in India for the remaining years of his life. In 1983 they moved to Sri Lanka, where he died at the age of ninety.

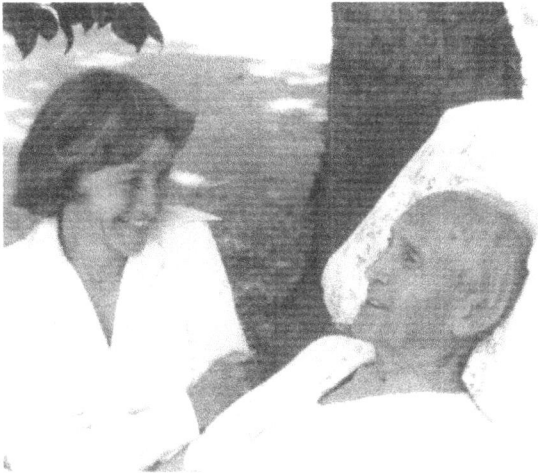

Sigfrid Knauer with his daughter Christina

Dr. Christina van Tellingen shares:

> Hendrik and I met Sigfrid Knauer in the spring/summer of 1980 after two intense years of study with Willi Sucher on the basics of anthroposophy. This was soon after Sigfrid Knauer suffered his stroke, which lamed his right side and made him aphasic. We started taking care of him together with Valery Morrison in August 1980 and continued till February 1981 in a house in Penryn, California, in the

foothills near Fair Oaks. It was rented by a group of his grateful patients.

Sigfrid Knauer was a special person who carried his discomfort with patience. His daughter, who visited him frequently, was always able to cheer him up. He was not always so easy to help, since he could mostly not simply say what he needed, such as, "I love fruit but will only eat ripe fruit." We had to add honey to his fruit for this reason sometimes, and that worked!

I was taking my USMLE exams during that time to be able to start an anthroposphic practice in California, since no one had taken up work as an anthroposophical physician in California after Sigfrid Knauer. By the end of our time together I was able to ask him my burning question: What is most essential when you are treating people anthroposophically? And he was able to answer over an hour's period of time and patience that the therapy is one whole, not to treat separate symptoms. That has accompanied me always in my life as a physician. Sigfrid Knauer stayed in the Penryn house till the summer of 1981, I believe.

Dr. Traute Lafrenz Page (1919–2023)

Born in Hamburg, Germany, Dr. Traute Lafrenz (not yet Page) studied at the Freie Gymnasium, a liberal-arts high school. Her revered teacher, Erna Stahl, introduced her to the idealistic thinking of the early 1800s, which was much in contrast with the Nazi doctrine promoted at the time. Through this teacher, Traute found the ideals that led her to read the *Philosophy of Freedom* by Rudolf Steiner and brought her to join the White Rose, a nonviolent group based in Munich which called for resistance against the Nazi regime. When Traute met Hans and Sophie Scholl and other members of the group, she felt inspired to become an active member. She helped the group print their very aggressive pamphlets against Nazi tyranny and brought them to Hamburg for distribution. Hans and Sophie Scholl were both tried and executed on February 22, 1943, having been found guilty of treason. Traute Lafrenz was arrested two months later. She was able to disguise the extent of her activities and was sentenced to one year in prison. Shortly after her release, she was rearrested because her full involvement in the Hamburg leaflet distribution had become known to the Gestapo:

> Her trial was finally set for April 1945, after which she probably would have been executed. Three days before the trial, however, the Allies liberated the town

where she was held prisoner, thereby saving her life. (Wikipedia entry for "The White Rose")

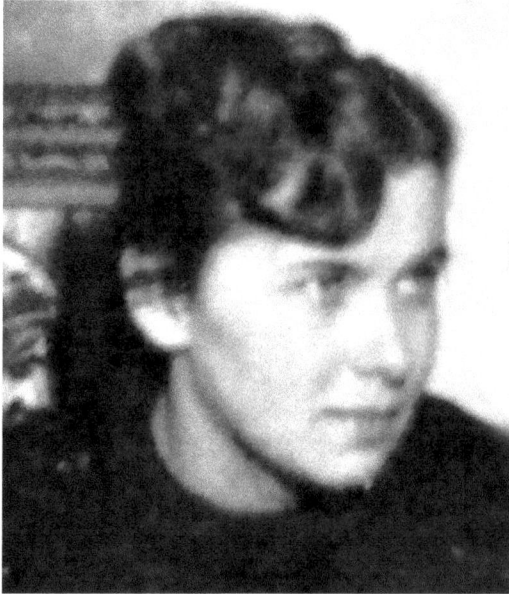

Traute Lafrenz

In 1947, Traute Lafrenz emigrated to the United States, invited by a Jewish childhood friend. She completed her medical training in San Francisco. During her residency, she met Vernon Page, who was also a doctor. They married in 1949 and had four children. After moving to Chicago, Dr. Traute Page was as a family doctor there for many years. She practiced anthroposophic medicine and supported the anthroposophic work locally and in the United States on a wide scale. In 1981, her vision was a strong force in the decision to move the administrative center of the Anthroposophical Society in America from New York City to the Midwest. She served as Co-General Secretary of the Society in the early 1990s.

Another facet of Dr. Page's work held close to her heart was the Esperanza School, a private therapeutic day school for students aged five to twenty-one with developmental disabilities. She was headmaster and medical director of the school for from 1972 to 1994.

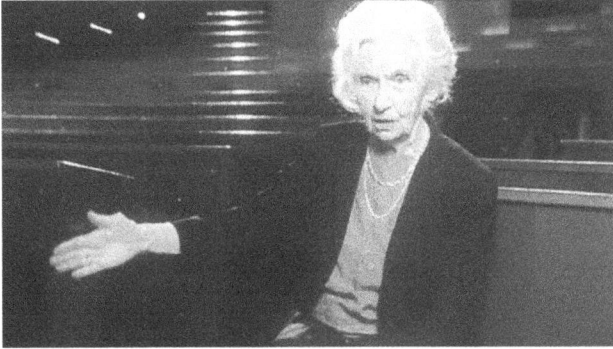

Dr. Traute Page

Dr. Traute Page celebrated her hundredth birthday in 2019, surrounded by her family in South Carolina. She was awarded the Order of Merit of the Federal Republic of Germany. Books have been written about her historic resistance against National Socialism. Many people realized that a true hero had laid the foundations of anthroposophic medicine in the Midwest.

In the Spring 2019 issue of *Being Human*, Barbara Richardson wrote for Traute's one-hundredth birthday:

Dear Traute! You had recently become the Director of Esperanza School when I first interviewed as a teacher there. You were an active, stylish woman who had a doctor's keen diagnostic eye (now I would say you are sanguine and mercurial with a bit of Mars to make it all happen!). As Director, you were able to speak with people from the Chicago Public

Schools, Department of Mental Health, as well as Chicago politicians. We had Mayor Harold Washington at our Oberufer Play one year. You cultivated their interest and financial support and we went from having a grade school to a whole range of life: birth to old age with therapies and workshops.

The parents and children loved you! You made the contacts with artists and teachers from Mexico, Germany, Emerson College and Waldorf Institute in Detroit.

As an anthroposophic physician it was wonderful to be with you in the Monday Study Group at the Rudolf Steiner Branch. You told us about the early days and the group who studied and helped make the little house on Grant Place a dignified home for the Society. With other groups we held seasonal festivals and regional conferences. You also brought several eurythmy troupes to Chicago. This culminated when the national Society moved from New York to Chicago. After many years on the General Council, you were asked to become General Secretary.

At one Council meeting at Fair Oaks [California] we were standing together on the sunny lawn at coffee break. I noticed you were unusually quiet and asked if something was wrong. You said this was the date Hans and Sophie died. You told me that you tried not to dwell on these things but there were certain dates when these memories were especially strong. When we had an outbreak of lice at Esperanza, you told me about your cell mate, a nun, who had very different spiritual views from yours. But the two of you had to pick the nits out of each other's hair and snap them between your thumbnails.

It was a great victory when a grant came through to build a big bathtub at Esperanza. It was the Therapy Room and was what passed for your office as well.

You and your therapeutic eurythmy colleague named it your "ether lab." It was such a great experience—an oil-dispersion bath, massage table with wonderful oils, and at the end you could do therapeutic eurythmy with the children. The parents loved it when their children came home smelling so nice—they knew their child had seen Dr. Page that day.

When people would call and beg for interviews for articles or television shows, you said they could come not to your lovely home and garden in the northern suburbs, but to the near west side in downtown Chicago. So, they would enter your Therapy Room and learn about anthroposophy, eurythmy and Waldorf education before you would answer their questions about your experiences.

One other heroic deed you did was make a home for your husband and four children. You tried to start a Waldorf school, but people seemed satisfied enough with their public school, so you took your children to the Christian Community through their growing up years. Advent is a very busy time, but you and your dedicated group of parents, priests, and musicians would perform all three Oberufer plays in one day. What strong people you were and what a strong foundation for anthroposophy you built in Chicago!

In the same issue of *Being Human,* Dr. Andrea Rentea shared these thoughts:

Traute Page was the family physician for our family starting in the 1950s in Chicago. She had a small but light-filled consultation room in her house. The first time I saw her I was a teenager and I had an episode of back pain. She greeted me coming from the garden with flowers in her hand. She promptly gave me my first anthroposophic injection—which worked! From her I first learned practical aspects of anthroposophical medicine, such as taking oral remedies, applying ointments, and administering injections. She made it all seem very doable.

The medical office was just one part of her extensive anthroposophical activity. At that time, in the absence of a "real" Waldorf school, she gathered together interested teachers and artists and did a "Waldorf Summer School." Also in the summers she visited the biodynamic farm of the Zinniker family in Wisconsin and made grape jam that our family really appreciated. In the winter, she invited everyone of the Christian Community to her house to sing the Kalevala songs. For years she led the Esperanza School; we visited her there and she demonstrated how she massaged the children to help heal them.

My husband and I are now practicing anthroposophical doctors in Chicago, her home town. We often feel that our activity here was made easier by her having laid the groundwork so many decades earlier. Thank you, Traute.

Therapeutic Education

The education for "children in need of soul care" was born out of Rudolf Steiner's Curative Education Course in the summer of 1924.* Among those who had asked Rudolf Steiner for help in this field was a parent couple from New York. They brought their nine-year-old boy, Sandroe, to the education course Rudolf Steiner gave in August 1923 at Ilkley, England. Both of his parents were early members of the Anthroposophical Society. His mother, Louise Mervin Roe-Stoughton, as Hilda Deigghton described, had been in 1908 a singing student of Mme. Ricardo in Berlin. It was Ms. Roe who introduced Mme. Ricardo to anthriposophy through Rudolf Steiner's book, *Theosophie*. Sandroe's father, Dr. Bradley Stoughton, a prominent metallurgy scientist, was a very supportive member of the St. Mark Group and had given public lectures on anthroposophy in New York.

After the conference in England, Sandroe, who was very restless and unable to attend school, was admitted to the Klinisch-Therapeutische Institut in Arlesheim, where Rudolf Steiner suggested treatment with anthroposophical remedies and therapeutic eurythmy. A pediatric ward was created and he was the first patient. A year later, under the leadership of

---

*   Rudolf Steiner, *Education for Special Needs: The Curative Education Course* (CW 317), Forest Row, UK: Rudolf Steiner Press, 2015.

47

Dr. Ita Wegman, this became the beginning of the Sonnen-hof home for children with special needs.

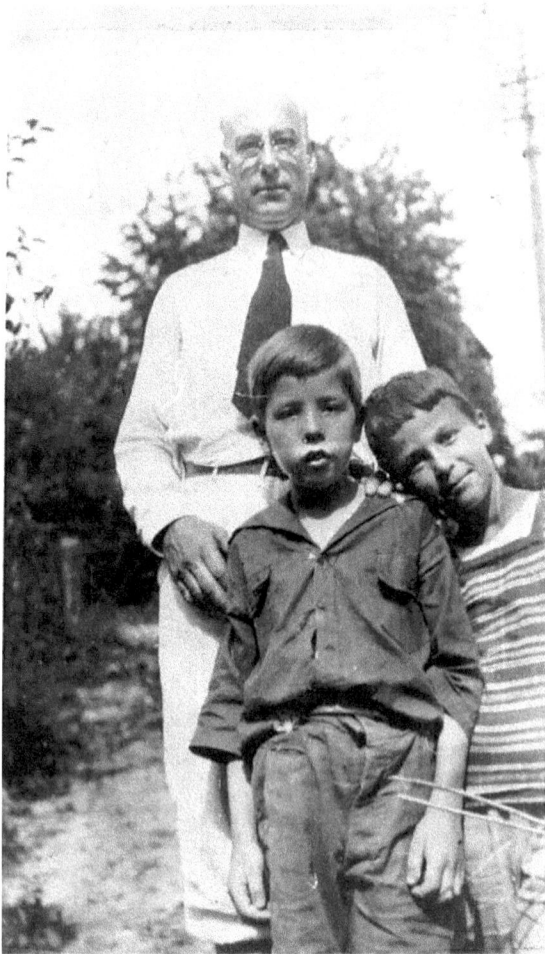

Sandroe, July 1924

In summer of 1924, Sandroe was the first child to be presented by Rudolf Steiner in the Curative Education Course, giving insights and direction for a new movement in therapeutic education. Over many years the boy grew up at the Sonnenhof. His parents visited him almost every year. During the second half of his life Sandroe lived at La Motta, a home Dr. Wegman had founded in Brissago in southern Switzerland.

One of the observations illuminated in the Curative Education Course was the boy's open-mouth breathing (characteristic of him also in later life). This, Rudolf Steiner elaborated, causes a prevalence of oxygen and lack of carbon dioxide, with consequences for his metabolism and constitution. During one of Sandroe's visits to his parents, an analysis of his breathing was performed by Dr. Karl Ernst Schaefer, head of the Physiological Research Institute in Connecticut, which confirmed exactly what Rudolf Steiner had described.*

❦

The first American home and school for children with special needs that worked out of anthroposophy was founded in 1938 at Lossing Manor by Gladys Barnett Hahn (1897–1994) and her husband William Hahn.

Gladys later wrote about the early history of the home (Ursel Pietzner, *The History of Beaver Run*):

> First there was Lossing Farm at Dover Plains, New York (1938–1950), with plenty of land, a large ancient house with six fireplaces, and a newly installed heating system that swallowed all of our money. Clara von Woedtke, a trained nurse from the Sonnenhof (Switzerland) worked with us for years. Dr. Christoph

---

* Wilhelm Uhlenhoff, *Die Kinder des Heilpädagogischen Kurses: Sechzehn Biographien: Krankheitsbilder und Lebenswege* (The children of the special education course: Sixteen biographies: Clinical pictures and life paths), Stuttgart: Freies Geistesleben, 2007.

Linder, and later Dr. Franz Winkler, came regularly (once a month) from New York to treat the children. Ten children were our limit: to us "small" was "beautiful." Neither of us was a "professional". We just wanted a family to whom we were "Uncle Bill and Auntie Gladys". Guitou Floch, a wild eight-year-old, and Aillinn Pusch, a seven-year-old deaf-mute, came. In summer, the children lived for blueberry picnics with a horse and an old wagon. In winter (and we had real winter) they lived for daily sledding. Johnnie, a five-year-old, stopped whatever he was doing—wherever he was without ever being told—everyday at five o'clock to go and get the milk pail and take it to the farmer at the barn. He was our afternoon clock.

We got the biodynamic gardening started, sold bushels of surplus vegetables every week on the local market, and had seventeen beehives at the peak of honey industry. It was a lovely place for the children.*

The paths that had led Gladys and Bill to Lossing Manor were unique. Gladys and Bill were both musicians from their younger days on. Around 1920, Gladys, trained as a concert pianist, had been the accompanist of Herbert Wilber Greene, a tenor and director of the first music conservatory at the newly opened Carnegie Hall. He had been brought to anthroposophy by Gracia Ricardo and held weekly readings of Rudolf Steiner's works at his summer school for music in Brookfield Center, Connecticut. Introduced by Mr. Greene to anthroposophy, Gladys was a participant in the summer school as well as her younger sister Ruth and William Hahn, a vocal student of Mr. Greene. All met in the early 1920s in the St. Mark Group, the anthroposophic branch that Mme.

---

*   Ursel Pietzner, *The History of Beaver Run: Thirty Years (1963–1993)*, Glenmoore, PA: Camphill Special Schools, 2004.

Ricardo and her friends had founded. Evolving from the St. Mark Group, Ralph Courtney formed the Threefold Commonwealth Group in 1923, with Gladys being one of its original members. It was the same group which three years later started Threefold Farm in Spring Valley.

Gladys sold her grand piano to afford her 1923 trip to Dornach, a bold decision which was characteristic of her. In Dornach she spoke with Rudolf Steiner and heard his lectures. She was invited to attend the August 1923 lecture conference in Penmaenmawr, Wales, and played the piano there for Rudolf Steiner and the conference participants. Destiny spoke when Gladys lost a lot of her hearing in 1924. She had to give up her musical career and instead took eurythmy training in Stuttgart, Germany, together with her sister, Ruth, and her friend, Elise Stolting. Soon she and Elise decided to pursue training in biodynamic agriculture, which they found on the farmland in eastern Germany (now Poland) where Count Carl von Kayserlingk had hosted the Agricultural Course by Rudolf Steiner two years earlier. Both friends returned to Spring Valley in 1927 to introduce biodynamic farming at the newly established Threefold Farm, the first such farm in America.

Another step in Gladys' life was her becoming committed to the care and education of children with handicaps. In the late 1920s or early 1930s she taught kindergarten at the Rudolf Steiner School in New York City and had her first experience with special needs children. Gladys went to Arlesheim near Dornach to study and learn about the care for children who need 'soul care' at the Sonnenhof under the guidance of Dr. Ita Wegman. She was also trained in therapeutic eurythmy there. After her return to the States,

Gladys worked for four years at the Devereux School for Exceptional Children in Philadelphia and was married to Bill Hahn, who had become a businessman. Their plan to set up a school to pursue therapeutic education as it was taught by Rudolf Steiner led them to find Lossing Manor. It was a beautiful estate, not far upstate from New York City.

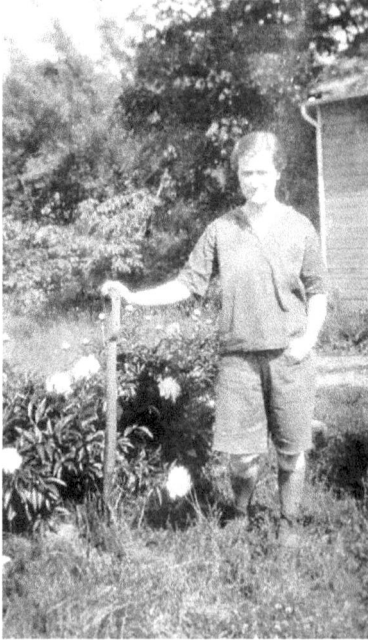

Gladys Barnett Hahn, 1927

After twelve years of operation Lossing Manor had matured. Gladys' niece Aillinn Pusch and other founding students had outgrown school age and the property had become too expensive. Aillinn went to California, where her parents had lived in Santa Barbara since 1949. The work at Lossing Manor ended in 1950. After two years of search and preparation, Gladys and Bill purchased an attractive farm in Copake named "Sunny Valley", not far upstate from

Lossing Manor, and in 1952 their work restarted. However, New York State regulations had become an obstacle for the work Gladys and Bill wanted to do. As a result, Sunny Valley was sold in 1954 and, with generous help from Alarik and Mabel Pew Myrin, an excellent place on the Myrin property in Downingtown in the countryside near Philadelphia was made ready for the school to operate.

Destiny spoke again when Bill Hahn suffered a severe stroke in 1958, leaving him bound to a wheelchair. The catastrophic situation opened the stage for the following amazing events. Gladys recalls:

> Suddenly, overnight, Bill had become a helpless invalid and I faced the appalling alternative of 'putting' him in an institution so that I could continue the school or putting the school into new hands so that I could nurse Bill. I gave myself a year to decide, and I suppose the gods were busy all that time.
>
> Finally, I wrote to Dr. Karl König, director of the Camphill Schools in Scotland. I had never seen him or any of the Camphill work, but knew his reputation. And I knew that the basis for his work and ours was the same: the philosophical and economical guidelines of Rudolf Steiner. I knew also that Dr. König had already sent coworkers from Aberdeen to start schools in Germany; perhaps he could do the same for America.
>
> And he did! So, in 1959 on the last day of August, with a famous heat wave hitting the Northeast, I met Janet McGavin at the New York dock. I loved her at once, because instead of asking, "Is it always so hot?" she said, "Tell me about the children!" By the time we reached Downingtown, we were good friends. There was just a week of "hand-over." Of course Janet made friends with the children at once.

This is Mrs. Toni Roothbert's story, which was unfolding at the same time:

> I think it's nothing short of a miracle how this place came to me. For twenty-five years I have been looking for a property suitable to develop on biodynamic lines. I looked at dozens of them in Vermont, in Massachusetts, in New York and Maine. I don't know how many times my husband saved me from buying a farm. Then one day I ran across a man in our neighborhood who wanted to grow food the organic way. And in the paper, there was an ad offering a farm in Millerton. So, we both were there. What a ramshackle place! Buildings practically unusable, decay all round. When I told the agent this was not the kind of place I was looking for, he offered me another which came on the market the day before. We all went to Copake. As we drove into the valley on a dirt road, the farm house and a small bungalow on our left, barns on our right, a sparkling creek, banks lined with willows following the road, white birches on the surrounding hills gleaming in the late afternoon sun, I knew "This is it".
>
> We suddenly saw two people standing in front of the farmhouse, I felt a stab in my heart. What do they want? They don't belong here, not that man in his dark city suit, nor the overdressed woman with jewelry dangling from wherever it could be hung. Yet they had just slipped a note under the door "Place sold". I turned my car round and went home. I felt miserable, and just about ready to give up all dreams of running a biodynamic holding.
>
> As I took my coat off, the phone rang and the Millerton agent said that he is still prepared to sell; the offer from the New York couple being too low. I negotiated the price for the 216-acre property on the telephone and asked whether the farm had a name. "Not

really," said the agent, "not now, but the couple who had it some years back called it Sunny Valley." I filled in the check for the down payment, and as I walked out into the night to the mailbox, I hardly knew anymore whether I was dreaming or waking.

Gladys continues:

While I was corresponding in 1959 with Dr. König, a letter came from a stranger, Mrs. Toni Roothbert living in Connecticut. She said she had just bought a farm in Copake, New York, and then while looking through an old Bio-dynamics Quarterly she noticed an advertisement: "Wanted: a Bio-dynamic farmer for Sunny Valley Farm, Copake." So, she was writing to reassure herself about the new property. Why had we sold it? Why had we left?

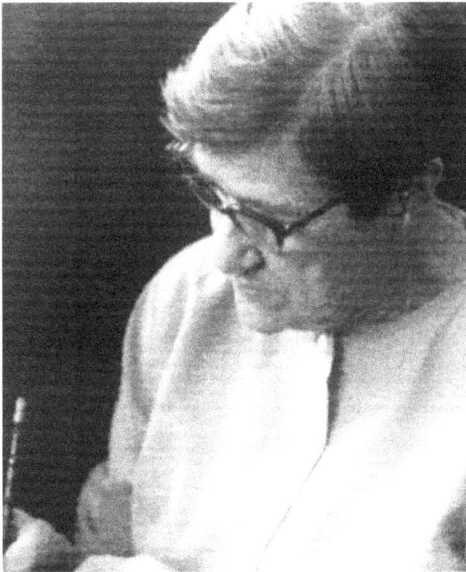

Gladys Barnett Hahn

She seemed so worried that I went to meet her in New York. My explanations were simple. New York State regulations made it impossible, Bill and I had thought, to continue a school there for small children. And our interest was centered in small children. With Mr. H.A.W. Myrin's generous help, we moved to Pennsylvania with its gentler regulations.

I told her of our present situation and of the expected arrival very shortly of coworkers to be sent by Karl König. "But then what are you and Mr. Hahn going to do?" she asked. "I don't know," I said, "I haven't begun on that problem yet." "Well!" she exclaimed, "Why don't you go right back to Sunny Valley Farm. I have no immediate plan for it. I've put a young man in the garage attic as a sort of caretaker. You shall be my guests, and you're welcome to go whenever you're ready."

In early September, therefore, after settling Janet in Downingtown, Bill and I returned to Copake. Toni Roothbert came often to see us. And who do you think arrived in summer 1960? Karl König! I remember how radiant he looked after he walked over the property. He had obviously been conversing with the gods throughout the entire morning. And now the gods became very busy. Mrs. Roothbert drove over the next day to meet Dr. König, and before the week had ended, offered to lease Sunny Valley to him—for a token fee—starting in Spring 1961, to build a Village for teenagers.

From this moment the gods must have gathered their own coworkers together and dispatched them in several directions. For people became active in New York City, for instance, to start financing the Village. Applications for young people began to reach Dr. König. I myself arranged to move to Spring Valley in 1961. Mrs. Roothbert felt nervous about her rather impetuous initiative and came over often to have me reassure her! And in May 1961 Carlo Pietzner arrived, sent by Dr. König to "take a look at Sunny Valley Farm."

Carlo was at this time engrossed in work at Glencraig, Northern Ireland. But apparently the gods knew him well and had him definitely in mind for the American project. I remember every detail of his visit. Janet had driven him up, and I invited a few towns-people for the evening, to hear directly from Carlo what a "Village" would be like and how it would relate to the town of Copake. Carlo was already identifying himself with it! It was this tiny gathering, squeezed into the tiny original "parlor" of what is now 'Orchard House' that worked out the name: Camphill Village.

In September 1961, Carlo Pietzner arrived to stay—Carlo and Ursel and their three children, and Renate Sachs and Mary Collins (soon to be Mary Elmquist). It was a tremendously exciting occasion for everyone! And a gloriously beautiful day. The sun was sparkling. The gods were smiling. Camphill Village began its history.

After the newcomers were accommodated in Sunny Valley, Gladys and Bill moved to Spring Valley for several years, where, besides the care for Bill, Gladys did therapeutic eurythmy and curative work with the students of the Green Meadow Waldorf School. In 1968, the Hahns returned to Copake, the property of which had been deeded by the Roothberts to Camphill the same year. Gladys saw the need of coworkers' children and started a nursery/kindergarten. She worked with Gerda von Jeetze and Natalie Brewer to begin the Rudolf Steiner Country School, the precursor of the Hawthorne Valley Waldorf School. During this time Bill became even more incapacitated and moved to a nursing home in Great Barrington, where he later died.

In the early 1970s, Gladys moved once more to Spring Valley and lived there with her sister Ruth for many years at the Fellowship Community. She taught students in the eurythmy training program, mentored teachers, and translated anthroposophic books. She and Ruth came to Copake (where Aillinn lived) for many visits, with Gladys often playing piano in the community hall. Gladys reached the age of ninety-seven.

❦

When the Camphill Village in Copake opened its doors in fall 1961, Aillinn was one of the first few villagers to arrive. She had already pioneered therapeutic education in the 1940s as a student of the Lossing Manor School. Born in 1933, deafness and developmental disabilities soon became obvious. Her American-born mother, Ruth Barnett Pusch, Gladys's younger sister, was a eurythmist. She and the German-born Hans Pusch had married in 1932. Hans had played major roles in Rudolf Steiner's Mystery Dramas at the Goetheanum. In 1924, he had been a participant in the Drama Course given by Rudolf Steiner. Ruth, Hans, and their two daughters lived in Dornach until their move to New York in 1939.

Aillinn grew up at Lossing Manor until the Pusch family moved to Santa Barbara, California, in 1949. By the time Aillinn arrived in Copake, the Puschs had returned to New York. She was now twenty-eight and would, from then on, spend her entire life, until the age of sixty-three, in Copake.

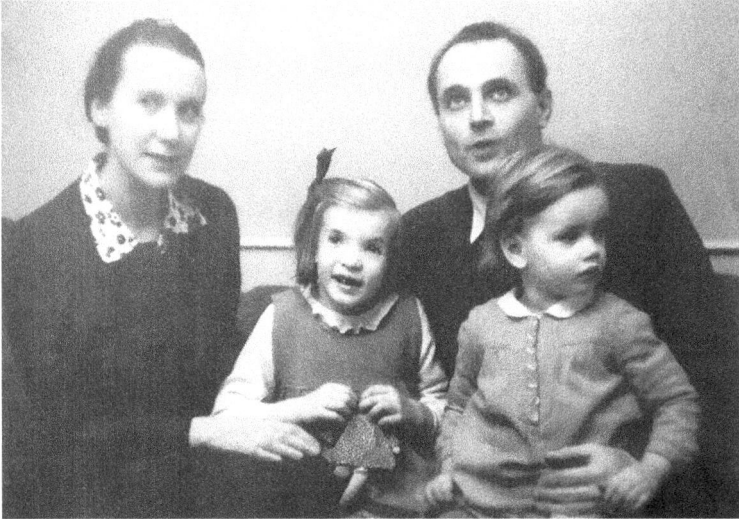

Ruth and Hans Pusch with Aillinn (left) and her younger sister

Penelope Baring, a pioneer Camphill coworker, wrote:

> I knew Ailinn very well, as she was my right hand in the kitchen for many, many years in Copake. I will never forget the twinkle in her eyes when she was up to something, like seeing me off to a meeting and then quickly baking up a batch of chocolate chip cookies for my children returning from school.
>
> I think that Ailinn did live for quite a few years with Hartmut and Gerda von Jeetze. She was very competent in the kitchen. When I moved to Tamarack House in 1978 she was part of an afternoon crew who worked alongside me to do cooking and housework for a household of between thirteen and fifteen in a given year. Aillinn could cook many meals independently and did so on Tuesdays and Wednesdays when I had meetings. I gave her the menu and she took it from there. Other days we worked together, she doing one part of a meal and I the rest. For me, she was a colleague. She had a great sense of humor and often

would point out things that tickled her funny bone, like an oddly shaped carrot or an amusing picture. She liked things to be "in order," occasionally too much so. Once I came home to find all the house plants had been given haircuts! She doted on my three children. The youngest, born in 1977, got full benefit. What I remember best are her dark, shining eyes. They could be either full of twinkling laughter or the warmest possible care.

Examples of How
the Legacy Developed Further

The work of the early founders of anthroposophically extended medicine and therapeutic education left a fruitful legacy. It had been accomplished by doctors, therapists, patients as well as helpers, artists, therapeutic teachers, children who needed special care, and their parents. Although by the time of Dr. Linder's death in 1964 there were less than ten anthroposophic doctors practicing in North America, new pathways had been opened for a younger generation, as will be mentioned here in a few examples.*

A major step was the creation of the Fellowship Community in Spring Valley, New York (today Chestnut Ridge), for the care of elderly people. Its legal basis became the "Rudolf Steiner Fellowship Foundation" which had already been set up as a charity in 1960 by Dr. Christoph Linder (and other anthroposophists, including Dr. Paul Scharff) to support the care of retired people in New York City. Dr. Scharff (1930–2014) had been one of the youngest in the group of doctors around Dr. Linder and was closely connected with his aims. When Nancy Laughlin, an anthroposophist and philanthropist, stepped forward with a generous donation, the

---

* Thorough descriptions of further developments were given in Henry Barnes, *Into the Heart's Land: A Century of Rudolf Steiner's Work in North America,* (Great Barrington, MA: SteinerBooks, 2013), as well as in Camphill literature and elsewhere.

Fellowship Community came into being through Paul, his wife Ann, and a group of coworkers and supporters in 1966.

Paul Scharff also felt indebted to the legacy of Dr. Ehrenfried Pfeiffer, who had furthered biodynamic farming in his later years in Spring Valley. Early in his life, Ehrenfried Pfeiffer had developed (under the direct guidance of Rudolf Steiner) the Crystallization Test, which today is widely used diagnostically in anthroposophic medicine and as a quality test for foods and in biodynamic farming.

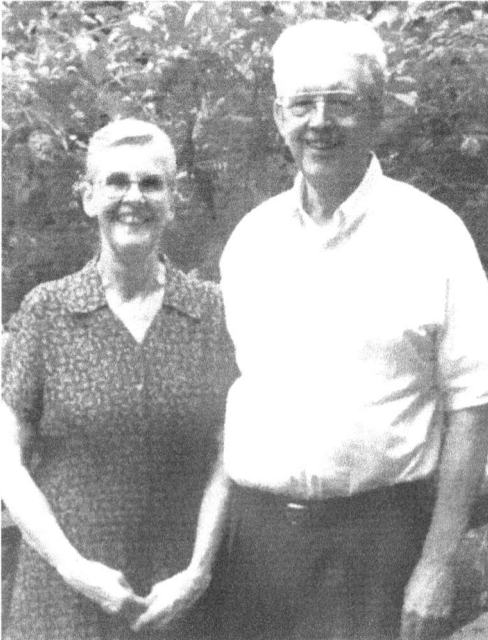

Ann and Paul Scharff

The services and initiatives brought forth by the Fellowship Community are comprised of: the retirement home (including advanced care), a general medical practice, the Otto Specht School for therapeutic education, publishing, biodynamic farming and gardening, and the hosting of medical conferences. As part of the Fellowship Community, Mercury Press published anthroposophical books for many years. In the mid-1970s Dr. Gerald Karnow, who had experienced Dr. Traute Page in his youth as a family doctor, joined the life of the Fellowship Community. He shared the medical practice with Dr. Scharff and continued it after Paul's death. The Fellowship Community continues to be a center of anthroposophic healing.

❦

In 1967, several anthroposophic physicians gathered in Spring Valley to form the Fellowship of Physicians, a working group recognized by the Anthroposophical Society in America and the Medical Section of the School of Spiritual Science at the Goetheanum. In the 1950s, Paul Scharff, Henry Williams, Franz Winkler, and Karl Ernst Schaefer had participated in weekend meetings with Christoph Linder. Traute Page came from Chicago; J. Herbert Fill and Percy Ryberg, both psychiatrists, joined. Dr. Fill was for a number of years head of the mental health system in New York City, then went into private practice. He was active in the Anthroposophical Society of America in many ways.

Henry (Hal) Williams, MD (1915–2002), a Quaker and a distinguished homeopathic physician practicing in Lancaster, Pennsylvania, had long been connected with anthroposophy. He was a steady participant and contributor in the anthroposophic doctors' work from the 1950s until his last years of life. Besides his busy practice, Dr. Williams kept visiting the new Camphill homes in Pennsylvania for many years.

Helen Zipperlen, editor of the booklet *Memories of the Beginning: Camphill in America 1961–1986,** wrote:

> Dr. Henry N. Williams—he seems to be everywhere—each of us must carry a vignette of him—encouraging us in sickness, delivering our babies, introducing a new person, a new idea—always a little mysterious, as though carrying a rainbow cloak woven from the gratitude of many people we do not know, but we depend on him as we have done for all these years.... Hal—you are between all the lines of this book!

Reflections by Christopher Schaefer on Karl Ernst Schaefer, M.D. (1912–1981):

> Karl Ernst was introduced by his wife, Ursula, to anthroposophy. He became intrigued with some of Steiner's statements about nitrogen, oxygen and carbon dioxide in the human organism. He told me that in an effort to disprove Steiner he did some simple experiments, being a physiologist, and found that Steiner's statements were correct, much to his surprise. This awoke a life-long interest in anthroposophy and in anthroposophic medicine.
>
> Most of Karl Ernst's research was connected to carbon dioxide since he had served as a doctor on a German submarine from 1940 to 1943. After the war he worked as an assistant professor at the University of Heidelberg on the potentially harmful effects of excess carbon dioxide in the atmosphere. While at the University of Heidelberg he was offered a job to serve as the head of the Physiology Branch of the Medical Research Division at the U.S. Naval Submarine Base in Groton, Connecticut. He accepted the job and moved to the U.S. in 1949 with Ursula and their four children.

---

* Helen Zipperlen (ed.), *Memories of the Beginning: Camphill in America (1961–1986)*.

He retained this job and position for the ensuing thirty years until his retirement about a year before his death. He initially settled in Charlestown, Rhode Island, in order to interact with Dr. Howard Laskey, an early practitioner of anthroposophic medicine. He subsequently moved to Old Lyme, Connecticut. He was an acknowledged international expert on respiratory and diving physiology in humans.

Karl Ernst was very interested in supporting anthroposophic medicine. Starting in 1977, he organized and helped to fund seminars for medical students and young doctors held at the High Mowing School in Wilton, New Hampshire. These seminars were led by Dr. Otto Wolff from Germany. Karl Ernst was also an active member of the Anthroposophical Society. Throughout his life he sought to bridge the gap between conventional scientific and medical research and anthroposophic medicine, and he is still remembered for these efforts as well as his seminal research on carbon dioxide.

Not having his own medical practice, Dr. Schaefer supported Dr. Laskey, who had also attended Dr. Linder's meetings, with his insights into Rudolf Steiner's teachings. In 1977, Dr. Schaefer started publishing a three-volume compilation, *A New Image of Man in Medicine,* with articles from notable anthroposophists and mainstream scientists. The compilation emphasizes the recovery of a holistic approach and "an effort to include the notion of the self and the individual biography in an understanding of health and illness." (Christopher Schaefer)

A group of medical students and young doctors had worked with Dr. Schaefer to be introduced to anthroposophy and anthroposophic medicine. Through the initiative of Dr.

Announcing 2 Therapeutic Conferences at Pine Hill School in Wilton N.H.

Knowledge of basic anthroposophical concepts essential.

I. The Four Members of Man

Physical body, ether body, astral body and ego.
JUNE 19 - 28, 1978
For medical students and physicians.
Anthroposophical concepts: Otto Wolff, M.D., Arlesheim, Switzerland
Related physiological data: K.E.Schaefer, M.D. , Old Lyme, Connecticut
Lectures by other physicians:

Philip Incao, M.D. — T. Page, M.D. — A. Rubinstein, M.D.
P. Scharff, M.D. — H. Williams, M.D. — B. von Zabern, M.D. and others

Tuition — $60. plus $5. contribution to the school.
For details write to: Dr. Karl E. Schaefer, 136 Neck Road, Old Lyme, Ct. 06371
Specify, please: sleeping bag arrangements or room
Prepare your own food (a group effort) or buy a meal

II. Seminar Introducing Rhythmical Treatment

according to Dr. I. Wegman and Dr. M. Hauschka
JUNE 28 - JULY 7, 1978
For persons with training or substantial experience in any field
of therapy, medical students and physicians.

Ms. I. Marbach, ''School for Artistic Therapy and Rhythmical Massage.''
Bad Boll, W. Germany, Dr. H. Williams and Dr. B. von Zabern
For details write to: Dr. B. von Zabern, Wilton, New Hampshire 03086

*Second Conference on Anthroposophically Extended Medicine, June
1978, sponsored by Dr. Karl Ernst Schaefer; first Conference on
Rhythmical Massage organized by Barbara von Zabern*

Schaefer, annual conferences for a wider audience of physicians and therapists were held in Wilton, New Hampshire starting in 1977. Led by Dr. Schaefer, the Physicians' Association for Anthroposophic Medicine (PAAM) was formed in the late 1970s. It was incorporated in 1982. The summer conferences continued first at the Pine Hill and High Mowing Waldorf Schools in Wilton, then in other locations with qualified teachers, mainly Dr. Otto Wolff. He was a prominent anthroposophic physician from Germany who had closely worked with Dr. Friedrich Husemann, one of the original medical doctors around Rudolf Steiner. The annual summer conferences with Dr. Wolff inspired and trained many young physicians and therapists who further pursued the spiritual approach to healing.

Since the early beginnings, therapeutic eurythmy, art therapies, and massage which followed Rudolf Steiner's teachings had been practiced under the guidance of the anthroposophic doctors. In 1978 and in the following years Rhythmical Massage conferences were held in different locations in the United States. They were first held by Irmgard Marbach, who with Dr. Margarethe Hauschka co-founded the School for Rhythmical Massage and Art Therapy in Bad Boll, Germany. A teaching curriculum in Rhythmical Massage was set up for training American therapists.

Anthroposophic nursing, therapeutic eurythmy, art, music, and other therapies took similar steps in working with the Medical Section at the Goetheanum. Formal training and certification were developed in the different fields, leading to the formation of an anthroposophic therapists' association, Artemisia, which later became an umbrella organization including PAAM and the Anthroposophic Health Association (AHA).

❦

In the 1980s, young anthroposophic physicians who belonged
to the Fellowship of Physicians and had met for years at the
PAAM conferences opened their practices, thinly spread out
over the eastern states, the Midwest, the West, and Canada.

Christina (Christa) van Tellingen, trained as a medical
doctor in the Netherlands, shares:

> My husband Hendrik, a physiotherapist, and I left
> Sigfrid Knauer's caretaking in order to take the
> anthroposophical doctor's course in Holland and
> then do my internship in California. Hendrik and I
> started the practice in Fair Oaks, California in July
> of 1982, because there was a small home for seven
> handicapped children there, run by Sunny Whalley.
> In September 1983, our team was enlarged with Cyn-
> thia and Harald Hoven and we founded the Friends
> of the Anthroposophical Medical Work Raphael
> Association, and moved to Raphael House, our own
> location in Fair Oaks. We tried to contribute to
> our local cultural heritage (the gold rush) by imple-
> menting a fundamental social law as formulated by
> Rudolf Steiner. We paid ourselves according to need
> and worked not each for ourselves but for the whole.
> We were able to keep that up as the Raphael Asso-
> ciation grew from four practitioners (doctor, phys-
> iotherapist, curative eurythmist, and gardener) to
> include eight therapists, a pharmacy, a home where
> people could stay to receive therapies and rest, and
> a garden that both provided the community with
> healthy biodynamic food through a CSA as well as
> garden therapy, altogether around twenty people.
>
> Hendrik and I were there till the beginning of 1998,
> when some of our special friends in Fair Oaks passed

away. We left to take up new challenges, which happened to be in the Netherlands.

Mark McKibben, an anthroposophic pharmacist, had worked for several years at the American Weleda and for two years in Germany at the WALA Company, which makes anthroposophic remedies. He also experienced, for a shorter time, the Ita Wegman-Klinik Pharmacy in Switzerland. In 1988, following an invitation by Christina van Tellingen, he started the Raphael Pharmacy in Fair Oaks, California, under the auspices of the Raphael Association. It produced WALA medicines as well as other anthroposophic remedies. Herbs for many preparations were grown in the Raphael Garden.

In 1996, after conversations with Ross and Andrea Rentea, Mark and his family moved to East Troy, Wisconsin, where Mark founded the Uriel Pharmacy. This has grown to be a major supplier of a great diversity of anthroposophic remedies (Based on a report by Mark McKibben).

After being trained in anthroposophically extended medicine in different places in Europe, Drs. Ross and Andrea Rentea started in 1983 the Paulina Medical Clinic in Chicago. Andrea had grown up there, having in her teens seen Dr. Traute Page as her family doctor. Years after Uriel Pharmacy had become established with their support, they founded in 2004, together with Dr. Mark Kamsler, True Botanica for "manufacturing supplements, remedies, and cosmetics, all based on Rudolf Steiner's indications that are specifically answering the real needs of our times" (from the True Botanica announcement letter). Connected with True Botanica is the Lili Kolisko Institute for Anthroposophic Medicine research laboratory.

Doctors Quentin and Molly McMullen, who were trained in anthroposophic medicine in Europe, opened in 1997 the Rudolf Steiner Health Center in Ann Arbor, Michigan. From the Steiner Health website, 2021:

> The Retreat Center is a historical building, just a short walk from downtown Ann Arbor. Originally built in 1916, the home is warm and spacious. The common spaces and art room are in the lower level and patient rooms and other therapy rooms are on the second and third floor (an elevator is available for those who need it). Steiner Health purchased the house in 2003 turning it into the first anthroposophical inpatient center in the United States.

The retreats offer courses of therapy to patients recovering from chronic illness, which are guided by the two internists. The full range of this anthroposophic medical approach provides treatment with natural and homeopathic remedies, diet, medicinal baths, rhythmical massage, therapeutic eurythmy, and different art therapies.

❦

Major steps in the development of anthroposophically extended medicine and therapeutic education were taken in Canada in the mid-1960s and in the decades to follow, which later included social therapy. Founded in 1968, the Toronto Waldorf School, after having started in a preliminary location, joyfully moved into its new building at Bathurst Street in 1973. Michaelhaven, an anthroposophic home for severely handicapped children, was established by Gabriele Zimmermann and a similar home by Christine Schuster, both near Toronto. There was a local group of therapists doing therapeutic eurythmy, music therapy, professional nursing, and therapeutic education. The author was privileged to visit the Toronto Waldorf School biannually from 1971 to 1982 as a school physician and to see children at the therapeutic homes. In the medicinal realm, Gerolf Zimmermann provided the distribution of Weleda preparations in Canada for a good number of years.

By 1981, a group inspired by the Fellowship Community in Spring Valley had formed in Toronto: Elisabeth Lebret, Christine Runge (who was a rhythmic massage therapist), Susan Samila, and other supporters pursued the goal to create an anthroposophic retirement community. The group grew to include a priest of the Christian Community and other anthroposophists experienced in nursing, architecture, financial planning, and other fields. Dr. Kenneth McAlister, who had a long-time connection with the Fellowship Community in Spring Valley, joined the cause bringing the vision of an anthroposophic medical center next to the retirement initiative.

The Hesperus Fellowship Community opened in 1987 with Elisabeth being its first resident!* In 1990, Kenneth accepted the executive leadership of Hesperus and oversaw its expansion, with a second Hesperus project opening its doors in 2011. Both retirement initiatives, consolidated into Hesperus Village, are on the same grounds as the Toronto Waldorf School, the Pegasus Medical Center and the Center of the Anthroposophical Society in Toronto.

Together with Dr. Werner Fabian (an anthroposophic family physician in Barre, 50 miles north of Toronto), Dr. McAlister founded in 1989 the Canadian Association of

---

* See the reminiscences shared by Susan Samila on the Hesperus Village website.

Anthroposophic Medicine, which connects anthroposophic physicians over the vast distances of Canada. He shares:

> In the 1990s I was very active "politically," founding various organizations with other holistic physicians to protect ourselves and lobby governments for a more enlightened view of what we were doing. Eventually we had a three-day conference with the College of Physicians and Surgeons in Ontario, our licensing body, at which I submitted a document for guidelines for practicing complementary medicine and it was accepted.

While PAAM had reached out to a wider audience, the Fellowship of Physicians, led by Dr. Scharff, carried the more esoteric work with the Medical Section at the Goetheanum. Due to the need for an entity to represent anthroposophic medicine and affirm its standards, the American College and Board of Anthroposophically-extended Medicine was formed in 1990. With the support of the College, in 2001 the PAAM developed guidelines and a curriculum for training physicians and other prescribing health care practicioners to be recognized to practice anthroposophic medicine. This effort was originally organized and carried by Dr. Alicia Landman-Reiner and more recently by Dr. Adam Blanning and others.

The medical conferences had grown to a stage where Dr. Michaela Glöckler, leader of the Medical Section of the Goetheanum School for Spiritual Science, came to America to attend the 1989 PAAM conference and to meet with the Fellowship of Physicians in Fair Oaks, California. Similar conferences repeated in the 1990s. Following a request made by Erk Schuchardt, the director of Weleda USA, and Alicia Landman-Reiner, on behalf of PAAM, since 2008 the International Postgraduate Medical Training (IPMT) conferences have traveled to different places in the United States as part of the PAAM curriculum. Through these conferences, webinars, and a three-year course of individual mentoring, many doctors and other licensed practitioners were trained and certified in anthroposophic medicine.*

These examples characterize the wider work that carried further what the pioneers of anthroposophically extended medicine had begun. Similarly, the beginnings of therapeutic education expanded with bold steps, including the care for adolescents and adults with special needs.

۞

Carlo Pietzner (1915–1986), who came with his family in 1961 to the new continent, was well prepared. Being trained at a well-known school for the arts and crafts, in 1937 he had joined the group of students around Dr. König in Vienna. Inspired by anthroposophy and the vision of Dr. König, these students became the founders of the Camphill Movement in Scotland. A good number of years later, Carlo Pietzner and Ursel Pietzner founded the Camphill Community in Glencraig, Northern Ireland in 1954.

When Carlo was asked to expand the work of Camphill to North America, the Camphill Village in Copake became his permanent home. Two years after Carlo's start at Copake, the Camphill School at Beaver Run (not far from Downingtown, Pennsylvania) came into existence through

---

* See Adam Blanning, MD, "Anthroposophical Medical Training in the United States"; in: *Der Merkurstab, Zeitschrift für Anthroposophische Medizin / Journal of Anthroposophic Medicine*, 2019, no. 3.

his initiative. With Carlo's help the Kimberton Hills Farm, the Triform Community for young adults in Upstate New York, and the Camphill Farm in Minnesota were founded.

Besides his work at Camphill, Carlo committed himself to the enhancement of anthroposophical activities at the local level as well as on a wider scale by serving on the Council of the Anthroposophical Society in America. He supported the forming of the new Section for Curative Education and Social Therapy as part of the Medical Section of the School for Spiritual Science at the Goetheanum. Under his leadership the Camphill Association of North America was formed in 1983. Being an artist, Carlo created paintings, stained-glass window art, and architectural designs of community halls and residences. He stayed in Copake till the end of his life.

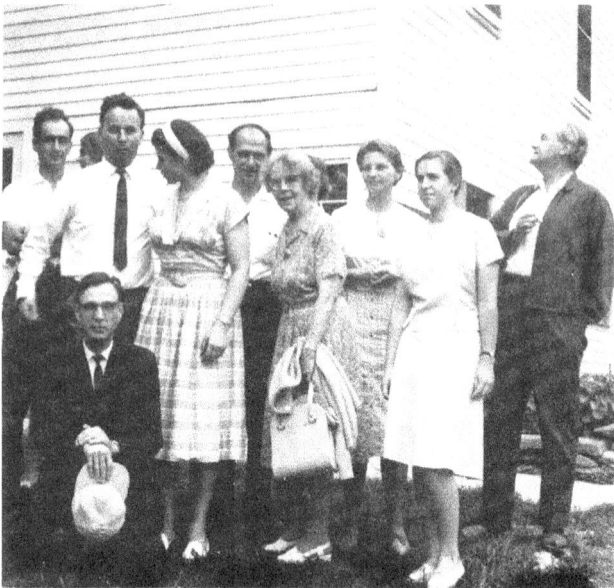

Carlo Pietzner (right) with Camphill coworkers
at a conference in Copake; Hartmut von Jeetze first left

Hartmut von Jeetze was part of a great group of devoted and vigorous coworkers who made the growth of Camphill possible. His roots originated in the very beginnings of biodynamic farming and therapeutic education based on anthroposophy.* His parents, Dorothea and Joachim von Jeetze, had attended the Agricultural Course given by Rudolf Steiner in 1924 in Koberwitz, Silesia, now part of Poland. In 1928 they made their sizeable mansion, Pilgramshain, not far from Koberwitz, available to Albrecht Strohschein, one of the initiators of Rudolf Steiner's Curative Education Course, his coworkers, and the cared-for children. In the same year Dr. König became part of the work at Pilgramshain, staying there for eight years.

1928 was also the year that Hartmut was born; he had known Dr. König, his wife, Tilla Maasberg König, and their children since childhood. After World War II, Hartmut and his wife, Gerda, followed Dr. König to Scotland, where they strongly contributed to the development of therapeutic education and biodynamic gardening. Both belonged to the founding group of the Camphill Village at Copake. After carrying the therapeutic social life and biodynamic farming work at Copake for many years, Hartmut and Gerda, with a team from Copake, founded the Camphill Farm in rural Minnesota. They stayed there for more than ten years, establishing a thriving community. In the years to follow Hartmut and Gerda would live in other Camphill communities in North America, sharing their knowledge and initiative. In their later

---

* See David Adams, "The Beginnings of Biodynamic Agriculture at Threefold Farm in Spring Valley, New York (and in the U.S.)," https://www.biodynamics.com/system/files/pdf/BeginningsOfBD @ThreefoldFarm.pdf.

years they settled in the new Camphill Ghent community for elderly people, located near Copake.

(&

Educational activities have been part of the development of the Camphill Movement in North America since the 1960s:

> With the spread of the Camphill Movement, professional training in curative education and social therapy became available in North America through what was then known as the 'Camphill Seminar', with courses at The Camphill School (formerly Camphill Special School) in Pennsylvania and at Camphill Village USA in Copake, New York. (Camphill Academy website)

By the year 2013, this training had evolved into the Camphill Academy, which allows students to earn a B.A. degree upon completion of the five-year program. As of 2021 there are now fifteen communities belonging to the Camphill Association in North America from coast to coast.

(&

Warmest thanks to Bernie Wolf, Penelope Baring, Marty Hunt, Wanda Root and other Camphill coworkers for generously sharing the literature, documentation, and remembrances which support this chapter and the one on Therapeutic Education.

Epilogue

A t any time, the true beginnings lie within ourselves. There are moments when we meet someone, often for the first time, that leave a lasting mark on our lives. One of these moments happened to me when, at one of the German doctors' conferences in 1963, I asked Dr. König whether I might possibly come to Scotland for six months as a volunteer. He looked at me with his concerned and powerful eyes and firmly said, "We will *make* it possible!" I had the distinct thankful feeling of being humbly small, while facing him. I would like to share a few more such encounters which connected me to the "beginnings" of this book.

Two years later, just days after my first arrival in America, I went to "Germantown", because I was curious to see the Weleda. I found Goodman's Pharmacy on the Upper East Side which to a German newcomer appeared as strange as Manhattan could be. The store looked ancient, all aged wood, but had a familiar balmy smell. There was a charming, "How may I help you?" from, as I learned, Christine's younger sister, Ursula. With my accent I asked whether they had a toothpaste? But rather than selling me the toothpaste, she wanted to know where I came from and, before I could say much, she went to the back of the store, from where Christine and Finbarr emerged to invite me for tea—the beginning of a lasting friendship.

After nine months of internship, when I had my first week-long break, I went to see the Midwest and the South. On my stopover in Chicago, Dr. Traute Page was kind to see me for a short visit. She sat on an easy chair, having one leg bandaged after vein surgery, speaking with me in her clear and comforting way with the steady gaze of what seemed to me to be steel-strong eyes. I realized much later that these eyes had once faced historic evil.

By the time I met Gladys and Bill Hahn that spring, Spring Valley was paradise compared to New York City. They had lived for a while in the old Gate House of the Fellowship Community, the same little house Barbara and I would move into three years later. Bill, sitting in a wheel chair, greeted me warmly. What struck me with Gladys was her festive joy and absolute confidence. She remembered my parents from around 1930 and immediately became an old friend. It took years for me to understand the enormity of the work she had fulfilled.

In the same year I headed by Greyhound to the Great West where I was able to visit Dr. Knauer. I remember him as a gentle person who gave me three-quarters of an hour of his precious time. We were in his small office at Sunset Boulevard in Hollywood, where the wall was covered with shelves of many medication bottles and containers. He was friendly, attentive, and frank. Much later in life I found, to my surprise, among my documents one signed by Dr. Knauer in 1935 in Berlin, stating that he had given me a smallpox vaccination.

In 1967, while I was back in Germany, Barbara and I made a beautiful trip to Brissago at the Lago Maggiore and visited La Motta. On one of our walks, a man who appeared to be in his fifties came toward us down the road and said, "I am Sandroe." After a little conversation he looked in a friendly way at Barbara and said slowly and thoughtfully, "You should wear a sweater. It is cool here in the evening."

When Barbara, our boys, and I immigrated in 1969 and the American soil still went up and down under our feet after a six-day cruise on the MS *Nieuw Amsterdam,* Ann and Paul Scharff stood waiting at the pier. It was a wonderful and warm welcome filled with hospitality to the new country we wanted to belong to.

A year later, I had the opportunity of meeting Dr. Winkler, whose memorial lecture for Dr. Linder I had heard a few years before. On his invitation we sat in the Café Geiger, close to Goodman's Pharmacy. Instead of the stern lecturer, there was a fatherly colleague as we talked about Vienna, from where he knew Dr. König, how they had met again in New York and about his concern for his New York practice which he wanted to give up—all in an atmosphere of friendship. In response to my question about patients who are not familiar with anthroposophy, he said, "All my patients are or become anthroposophists."

Because Dr. Linder had already passed in 1964, I was unable to meet him. But my parents knew him well from the late 1920s through the St. Mark Group, the Weleda work, and the eurythmy. Irma Gebauer, my mother, worked from 1930–1931 as a therapeutic eurythmist in Dr. Linder's office, sent by Dr. Wegman. I often heard my parents speak about him and other friends from New York when I was a child. When my father, Arthur von Zabern, returned to Europe in 1932, he was invited on a luxury liner trip by Mme. Ricardo, his Weleda chief. He remembered that when he, being a young man, and Mme. Ricardo, who had a majestic appearance, had to climb the steep ship stairways, Madame would say from time to time, "Arthur, give me a push!" Thirty years later, he visited Dr. Linder who was being treated for his stroke at the Ita Wegman-Klinik. Christoph complained not so much about his health but about, as he believed, not having fulfilled his task of establishing anthroposophic medicine in America enough, a humble and noble complaint.

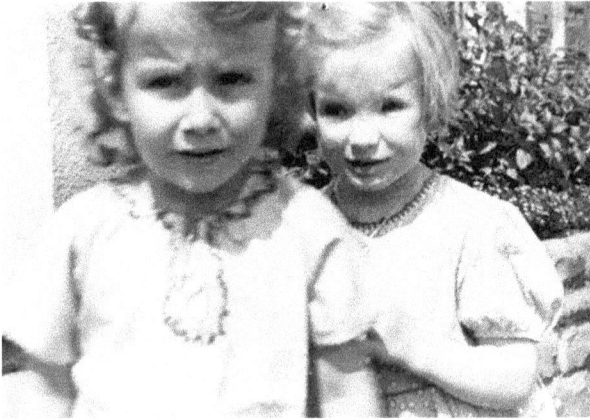

Aillinn in 1937

Aillinn and I were both born in 1933. She even was a guest at my first birthday party in Arlesheim. She and her parents visited us a few years later in Stuttgart, which I remember well. She was "wild," wanting all my toys and tossing them around, which made me unhappy ("Understand me!" was the cry of her soul—reminiscent of Helen Keller). Many years later, when I met Aillinn again, she was a warmhearted and perceptive personality with a fine sense of humor, who loved taking care of little children.

Every one of these moments of remembrance, which stand for many others, are seeds of new purposes and commitments. They are the real story.

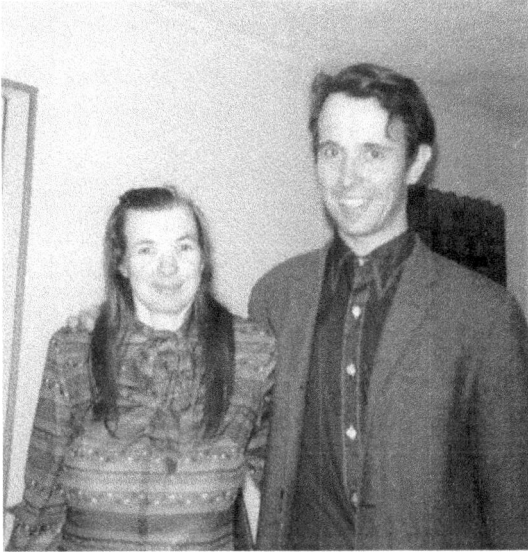

Aillinn in 1974

Books by Bertram von Zabern

Compendium for the Remedial Treatment of Children, Adolescents and Adults in Need of Soul Care: Experiences and Indications from Anthroposophic Therapy

Organic Physics: In Search of a Science of Life

Warmth: Living Element and Healing Substance

Angelus Silesius: Cherubinic Wanderer: Verses Selected and Translated

The Rosicrucian Stream in the Live of Those Touched by It

All titles available from www.amazon.com

www.ingramcontent.com/pod-product-compliance
Lightning Source LLC
LaVergne TN
LVHW010318070426
835511LV00026B/3492